HOME BIRTH

I would like to dedicate this edition to
Beverley Beech and all the dedicated AIMS team
to whom women who want freedom about
the way they give birth owe so much.

NICKY WESSON

Nicky Wesson has a long-standing interest in childbirth, both current and historical. She has been an antenatal outreach teacher, chair of her local Maternity Services Liason Committee and founded the West London Homebirth support group almost 20 years ago. She has attended many births – both at home and in hospital – and has six children.

She has written six books on pregnancy, childbirth and alternative therapies including *Alternative Maternity, Home Birth, Morning Sickness, Labour Pain* and *Alternative Infertility Treatments*.

Nicky is a medical herbalist living and practising near Hampton Court. She has an especial interest in working with fertility, pregnancy and childbirth and children.

HOME BIRTH

A PRACTICAL GUIDE

pinter & martin

PINTER & MARTIN

Home Birth: A Practical Guide

First published by Macdonald Optima 1990
This 4th edition published by Pinter & Martin Ltd 2006

ISBN-10: 1-905177-06-2
ISBN-13: 978-1-905177-06-6

British Library Cataloguing-in-Publication Data
A catalogue record for this book is available from the British Library.

Set in Agenda

Printed and bound in Great Britain by
Creative Print & Design, Ebbw Vale, Wales, UK.

Pinter & Martin Ltd
6 Effra Parade
London SW2 1PS

www.pinterandmartin.com

contents

preface to the fourth edition

It has been very interesting to look at home birth again – seventeen years after writing the first edition of this book and nearly twenty years after starting one of the country's first home birth support group. It is fascinating to discover that the research evidence which was rejected by the medical establishment then has now been embraced and endorsed by NICE (the National Institute for Health and Clinical Excellence). Home birth is now recognised to the extent that NHS Direct[1] can state that 'studies have shown that it is equally safe (for healthy women) to be attended by midwives in the comfort of your own home as to have your baby in hospital. If you do not plan to have an epidural and want to be sure of having a midwife with you during your labour, home birth is a recommended choice.'

The irony is that now the struggle to establish the safety of home birth is won, the right to be attended by a midwife in the comfort of your own home hangs by a thread.

Of course the concept of home birth being safe or safer than hospital birth has not been universally accepted. While I was researching this edition, I rejoined my home birth support group which continues to flourish. There I heard about the negative ways in which women's request for a home birth had been greeted by their doctors as well as by friends and relations, even though choosing to have a baby at home is less uncommon these days. Many of these women needed to be determined in order to get their booking, and I know that many others have asked to have their babies at home and been deterred. The Association for Improvements in the Maternity Services, who have been working with dedication for over forty years to help women with birth, have a list of reasons why women have been refused a home birth that would be almost laughable if it didn't matter so much.

However, possibly a bigger problem, because of the uncertainty of provision and distress it causes, is the current situation, whereby a woman can obtain a home birth booking comparatively easily but then be told late in her pregnancy that it may not be possible to provide her with a midwife when she goes into labour because of staff shortages. This is because there is no longer a legal obligation to supply a midwife for home birth and Health Trusts up and down the country do not feel obliged to guarantee a home birth service. Provision rather than demand dictates whether women can have their babies at home, so that in some areas one in seven babies will be born into their own homes, while in others fewer than one women in two hundred has a home birth. Equally, in some areas over half the first-time mothers booked to give birth at home were transferred to hospital during labour[2] and in some areas fewer than 2 per cent of women for whom it was not a first baby were transferred. Some need for transfer is undeniable, but other transfers may reflect lack of confidence among midwives or lack of enthusiasm for providing an efficient home birth service, so that women are compelled to give birth in hospital against their wishes.

In many instances the lack of support for home birth comes from midwives who do not feel confident about assisting birth away from the comfort of the hospital setting which provides them with easy access to help and moral support. I do not underestimate the responsibility of attending home birth as a midwife – it is a matter of life and potentially death. I think that it is easy to take a midwife's competence for granted, not taking her doubts and feelings into consideration. The Nursing and Midwifery Council has recently made it clear that it is a midwife's duty to have or acquire the skills to undertake home births with competence. With the current Government backing to encourage home birth,[3] the obligation must lie heavily on providers to ensure that midwives are trained to be confident about home birth.

When I was almost at the end of writing this edition, NICE brought out draft guidelines for intrapartum (labour) care. NICE is an independent organisation that considers the evidence for interventions in health provision – NHS professionals should be guided by its findings. Their evidence on many issues will prove welcome to women keen to give birth with as little intervention as possible. These include wider parameters of low-risk, particularly with regard to low haemoglobin, premature rupture of membranes, electronic fetal monitoring in labour, upright positions in labour, support for a physiological third stage of labour in low-risk women and their recommendation over provision to be made for annual updates for midwives on resuscitation for the newborn. I would take issue with their tentative suggestion that there may be a higher risk of perinatal mortality in babies born at home – James Hughes of the Institute for Ethics and Emerging Technologies, who has analysed 33 studies of home birth in his Changesurfer consultancy, found only one study that had this finding. It seems to me that it would take only a few women to decide to give birth at home to a child that is known to have no chance of survival at home, for these figures to be misleading.

This leads me to believe that the responsibility of individual women to insist on provision for birth at home, and its consequent rewards, is greater than ever. Now that we have the evidence together with official backing, it is only lack of vocal consumer demand that holds us back from a home birth for every woman that wants one. I believe that women have responsibility to ensure that they are fit for labour, to be well-informed and to ensure that the authorities provide them with confident midwives to help them have their babies at home. The support available to help them do this is greater than ever, and includes over seventy UK home birth support groups, thoroughly researched internet support and even government backing. If seen as part of a bigger picture and that your stand is not just for you but also other women, we can return the home birth rate to one that reflects desires rather than provision. There is a real opportunity to restore home birth to the norm if we only seize the chance.

Nicky Wesson
September 2006

acknowledgements

I would like to thank all the people who helped me to write this book by sharing their experiences of home birth. I am most grateful for the huge amount of support and encouragement I have been given. Women who have had babies at home are keen that others should share the same advantages. The efforts of the following, together with many others who are fostering home birth, should mean that more women will enjoy giving birth at home too: Hilary Adam, Iain Anderson, Gulperi Ataco, Gwen Atwood, Jan Ayres, Paula Ayres, Beverley Beech, Jo Bhatti, Charlotte Burns, Sam Cairns, Deborah Collier, Linda Collier, Karen Condon, Mary Cooper, E.M. Court, Marie Coveney, Tricia Coyne, Liz Crawley, Mary Davies, Joan Davis, Sally Dean, Caroline Dixon, Sara Drake, Nadine Edwards, Caroline Flint, Debra Flynn, Annie Francis, Catherine Gash, Sue Gerryts, Jill Gingell, Oona Gleeson, Harriet Griffey, Carole Guyette, Linda Hartley, Juliet Harwood, Heather Heales, Vanessa Helps, Jan Hibbert, Valerie Hill, Angela Horn, Miranda Hourihane, Adele Hulse, Hazel Johnston, Bruce and Juliet Leith, Barbara Lewis, Lucy McAteer, Angie Mindel, Christine Mole, Catherine Morgan, Jackie Murphy, Joanne Nicholds, Dorothy Norris, Joanna O'Brien, Jenny O'Keefe, Sue Paddick, C. Parker-Jones, Karen Parkinson, Kim Pearl, Elisa and Ben Peterson, Sylvie Price, Wendy Primmer, David Raitt, Jackie Reay, Lesley Redmond, Linda Riley, Helen Roberts, Jan Rumball, Jane Sandall, Catherine Seagar, Alison Smith, Kate Smith, Sally Smith, Stacia Smales Hill, Gayle Stanley, Catherine Sykes, Pat Taylor, Marjorie Tew, Alicia Thom, Twickenham Home Birth Support Group, Brenda van der Kooy, Lindsay Williams, Deborah Wilson, Jane Worden, Naomi Zair.

I would especially like to thank Christine Grabowska, who has been an unfailing source of inspiration and information. In many ways this book is her book as well.

preface

While doing my own research into the facts about home birth I discovered that there was generally a great deal of ignorance about the subject. This centred on the erroneous beliefs that a woman did not have the right to deliver a baby at home, that you had to be accepted by a doctor and that it was the safest way to have a baby in hospital. I also found that battling against the consensus of medical and social disapproval, while knowing only a very few people who had had babies in their homes, was a lonely and dispiriting process.

I myself felt the need for a book on the subject which would dispel the myths and give me practical information on all aspects of giving birth at home – and most importantly which would illustrate this information with the case histories of women who had battled through and won. I felt that women needed the courage that knowing others had succeeded against the odds, even when their pregnancies or labours were not routine, would bring. Such talk of battle and courage may seem an overstatement until you yourself encounter some of the ferocious opposition that asking for a home birth can arouse. For reasons which I will examine, the whole issue is astonishingly emotive and I hope that this book will provide an effective weapon against the huge weight of propaganda for the other side.

1 introduction

I decided to write this book as a result of my own experiences of home birth. My conviction that home birth was superior to a hospital delivery was prompted by my good fortune in attending two births at home, one planned and the other accidental. I could not help comparing these births, even though neither went according to plan, with the births of my own three children. These were high-tech deliveries with a great deal of intervention in a large London maternity hospital. I felt that submitting to that style of delivery in an alien environment, surrounded by strangers, had required a lot of courage, and the experiences had left me feeling angry and resentful and unable to look back on the events with pride. The births did not seem to be my achievement and I preferred not to think about them.

In contrast, while helping at the planned home birth I was struck by how very different the atmosphere, and expectations, were. I found that events were controlled, in so far as labour can be controlled, by the parents rather than the midwives. There was no doctor there, there was nothing to prevent my friend doing exactly as she wished, the midwives were well-known to her, her husband had an active part to play, all the comforts of her home were available to her – in fact the whole event felt much more relaxed and uninhibited than I had believed possible.

So impressive were these experiences, and so superior were they to even a sympathetic low intervention hospital delivery that I was also fortunate enough to attend around the same time, that when I became pregnant for the fourth time I was determined to have the baby at home. Determined is the right word, because obtaining a home birth proved to be a battle and I needed all my determination to hold out for what I wanted. Since then I have found that a really alarmist reaction to such a request can be considered normal, but at that time I was not really prepared for the wave of shock and opposition it would cause. My doctor was appalled and took 40 minutes of surgery time to tell me so; the director of the community midwives visited me and spent an hour and a half trying to dissuade me; and the reaction of my family and most of my friends was not much better. Admittedly I had had a Caesarean section with my second child, and that definitely puts you in the high-risk category as far as obstetrics is concerned. However I felt so bad about the hospital births that I no longer felt that I merely wouldn't agree to have the baby in hospital, but that I couldn't.

In an attempt to make me agree to a hospital delivery, increasing concessions were offered, but this only made me feel even more isolated and persecuted. I felt little consideration was taken of the fact that I was pregnant, and the weeks passed with my feeling depressed and lonely. I did get my booking with the community midwives, but they did not express any enthusiasm about the idea of the home delivery and I did not feel that I could trust them not to find some hidden complication at the last minute. Elaborate arrangements were made for the eventuality of something going wrong, including the need for me to be transferred to the third most distant hospital in case of an emergency in order to concur with health authority boundaries. I felt that I could not admit to any doubts about my decision, or tell anyone of anything that seemed amiss with the pregnancy. Then a slight rise in blood pressure was pounced on with zeal, and I had duplicated care from midwives and GP; neither was prepared to relinquish their checks, and whereas I would have appreciated this attention first time around it was far from convenient when I already had three children.

Because of this lack of trust I spent quite some time searching for a midwife, and at 36 weeks of pregnancy I found exactly the right person. Gwen worked independently, which meant paying for her services, but I feel they were worth every penny. She was enthusiastic about the birth, calm about the prospect of complications, took all the weight of worrying about the authorities off my shoulders and freed me to enjoy my pregnancy at last. I felt as if I had rolled into a feather bed, and the baby started to grow well.

Far too soon, although in fact five days late, I went quietly into labour on Sunday afternoon while having a barbecue with friends. I spent part of the evening scraping paint and getting the children into bed. At 9.30, when they were all settled, I had a bath and could admit I definitely was in labour. At 10.30 I rang Gwen and was able to let her in and make raspberry leaf tea for us. I felt completely in control and relaxed about what was happening. I got on with icing a birthday cake and stopped for the contractions, leaning over a bookcase. I was able to write down the time of the contractions while my husband sat on the sofa working. At 12.00 the waters went and by 12.30 Octavia was born on to the bedroom floor, at least six hours before I had expected her. We waited for the placenta to be delivered and then we had a candlelit bath together. Both of us in clean nighties, we went back to the bedroom and slept briefly before being woken by a glorious dawn. I was able to show my earliest-rising son the overnight arrival and treasure the memory of his excited, incredulous and happy expression. I then rang my mother and went back to bed to enjoy showing the baby to the others and getting to know her myself. Over the next few days we rested together happily and without disturbance before picking up the threads of a hectic family life.

There was nothing about hospital delivery that I missed and it was wonderful having Octavia join us so easily. And for the rest of the family it meant there were no long hauls to the hospital to meet the baby in alien surroundings, poorly equipped for forging new family bonds.

This was a labour I could look back on with pride, not resentment. It had gone the way I wanted; I neither received nor required any intervention, drugs or instruments; I did not have to decide when to go to hospital; no one else was giving birth at the same time; the event was completely special and unique but none the less quite matter of fact and without fuss; I felt no inhibition or tension; there was no one there that I did not want or did not know. As far as the children were concerned there was no break in routine – Octavia was simply not there one day and had arrived the next. She grew up to be an especially sunny, relaxed and happy little girl – qualities often noted by other mothers in their home-birth children. This suggests that being born at home may have lifelong advantages for the child as well as the mother, who never forgets her children's birth no matter how long she lives.

2 history

Internationally and historically, home birth is customary. It still is largely the norm in all but the developed countries, and even in them the switch to almost 100 per cent hospital births is comparatively recent.

In the 19th century giving birth within an institution was both unpopular and dangerous. At that time going into a hospital, generally a charitable lying-in hospital, greatly increased your chance of contracting puerperal sepsis (puerperal fever). This is a disease of childbirth which is caused by infection developing in the raw area of the uterus left by the detached placenta; it starts a few days after the birth, gives rise to fever and fits, and is eventually fatal. Without any idea of the way it was spread by medical attendants, or any cure, it meant that between 2 and 14 women per thousand died after giving birth at this time, and although the mortality rate fell it remained a killer until the 1930s, when antibiotics (sulphonamides) were discovered.

The hazards of hospital birth were clearly appreciated by Florence Nightingale, who commented in 1871 that:

> It must be admitted, at the very outset of this enquiry that midwifery statistics are in a very unsatisfactory condition. . . . But with all their defects, midwifery statistics point to one truth; namely that there is a large amount of preventable mortality in midwifery practice, and that, as a general rule the mortality is far, far greater in lying-in hospitals than among women lying in at home.

However, the number of women exposed to the hazards of the lying-in hospitals was comparatively small. By 1890 the percentage of women delivering in such hospitals and in workhouse infirmaries was 1 per cent, an almost exact reversal of the situation there was nearly 100 years later, when the percentage of births at home was around 1 per cent.

The reasons for this change were analysed in Rona Campbell and Alison MacFarlane's excellent booklet *Where To Be Born.*[4] Outlined briefly, the reasons for the increase in institutional birth largely hinge around safety, the assumption being that the fall in perinatal mortality was a result of the increase in hospital delivery. This assumption will be questioned in Chapter 4.

The change-over was initiated by the Notification of Birth Acts of 1907 and 1915, which gave grants to local authorities in order to provide antenatal visits to women in their homes, home helps, maternity centres with antenatal and infant welfare clinics and the provision of inpatient beds.

By 1917-18 the First World War had halted building schemes and towns became overcrowded. The Local Government Board's Annual Report 'emphasised the need for maternity homes for women who could not safely or conveniently be confined in their own homes'. Consequently the numbers of hospital beds steadily increased, although they were mainly intended for women who had complications of pregnancy or labour.

As a result, by 1927, when the first statistics about live births and their place of delivery were collected, 15 per cent of them were noted to have taken place in institutions. This category included maternity homes and Poor Law institutions as well as hospitals. By 1932 this figure had risen to 24 per cent, and by 1937, ten years after the first statistics were available, it had more than doubled to 34.8 per cent.

In 1936 the official view of the British Medical Association was that 'All the available evidence demonstrates that normal confinements, and those which show only a minor departure from the normal, can more safely be conducted at home than in hospital', a view which the evidence shows should still hold today. They also felt at that time that 'pregnancy and childbirth is a natural physiological event, even though it is one involving complex, delicate and important processes. Departures from the normal occur in a small proportion of cases'.

By 1944 the Royal College of Obstetricians and Gynaecologists were recommending that there should be provision for 70 per cent of births to take place in hospital. In 1948 the National Health Service was formed, and this encouraged more women to have their babies in hospital, partly because women could now get their antenatal care from their GPs and hospital clinics, and partly because the municipal community clinics, hitherto the only source of free antenatal care, were unable to treat complications or disease. Moreover, attending the GP or hospital clinic increased the chance of receiving continuity of care.

A truly fascinating account of the work of district midwives in the period 1948-72 is given by Julia Allison in the William Power Memorial Lecture of 1991.[5]

In investigating the work of midwives in the Nottingham City area, she borrowed more than 300 birth registers from retired and working midwives, containing details of more than 3,500 home births. Midwives at this time were enormously busy, delivering as many as 200 births each per annum. They were employed by the local authority, and practised almost totally independently of doctors – 95 per cent of births at home being conducted by district or pupil midwives, with no doctor in attendance.

District midwives attended all planned and unplanned home births, obstetric emergencies and babies born before arrival at hospital. They provided all the postnatal care, as well as attending antenatal clinics. They ran motherhood classes, were responsible for sterilising their equipment, replenishing their drug supplies and updating their records – as well as providing 24-hour labour and emergency cover.

Although their feet can barely have touched the ground, their record of delivering babies was extremely impressive. Allison cites the example of two midwives working as a team in March 1-7 1958 who delivered twelve babies between them during the week – three on the same day.

Picking at random a team of two newly qualified midwives working in the same year, she found that they attended all of their 233 clients in labour, coping alone with 23 first-time mothers, 27 grande multiparas (women who had had five babies or more who are held to be at greater risk of complications), a twin pregnancy, three breech presentations, many premature and postmature pregnancies and two women who had previously had ectopic pregnancies.

They had no stillbirths or maternal deaths. Two women had postpartum haemorrhages which they treated successfully at home. A GP attended four of the births, although all the babies were actually delivered by the two midwives.

At the time about 50 per cent of pregnant women had home births although less than half that percentage would fit into the low risk category that would be considered eligible for birth at home today. The transfer rate was less than one woman per midwife per year.

Intriguingly, both the mortality rate for babies less than 5 lb 8 oz in weight and the stillbirth rate were consistently and substantially lower at home, even though the births at home occurred in the areas of the city where the most socially disadvantaged were grouped. Premature and growth-retarded babies survived better in their homes than they did if they were born in hospital. Of babies weighing less than 5 lb 8 oz in weight who were born at home, whether or not it was their intended place of birth, 9 per cent died whether or not they were transferred to hospital. 17 per cent of those born in hospital died. The very sickest babies who were bound to die were kept at home in recognition of the fact that their mothers preferred to nurse them in the loving confines of their family. The mortality rate for both hospital and home-born babies declined at the same rate over the years.

Babies of all weights survived at a greater rate if born at home and this was recognised by the Medical Officer of Health for Nottingham in a 1953 memorandum which stated, 'It has been found with proper selection of cases and by the provision of specialised nursing care and equipment, premature babies born at home generally do better to remain there.'

Julia Allison shows that midwives delivering babies at home were capable of providing better outcomes for mothers and babies than is currently the case for women going into hospital. They clearly could deliver babies that are deemed to be at very high risk of encountering problems, e.g. breech, twins, and the premature babies who nowadays are considered to be safe only in a doctor's hands. True, modern midwives are not experienced in delivering such babies, or often any others at home. But the capability is theirs if they can only reclaim it. With the official recognition of the safety of home birth and an increase in the numbers of babies being born into their homes, perhaps we will be able to return to a time when childbirth was a happier experience for mothers and babies.

The new NHS regulations meant that a doctor rather than a midwife was the first point of contact for a pregnant woman;

women had direct access to a doctor instead of access to the doctor being via a midwife. This had longlasting effects on the degree of control which midwives had over maternity care. Hospital births doubled in number as GPs, who then had (and still have) a financial interest in maternity care, took over from the midwives. Midwives now became 'maternity nurses' when they attended deliveries where there was a supervising doctor present. As their status declined, so did the number of home births.

However this was not the only reason for the increase in hospital births in the 1940s. In a national survey of all births occurring in a week in 1946, it was found that 53.7 per cent of births were taking place in hospital. The Second World War was in some part responsible; as one woman who gave birth after the war commented:

> **"Women wanted babies in hospital because it meant you did not have to provide food out of your rations, someone else would do the laundry – things were very scarce. It was for reasons of housekeeping not safety that we wanted to go in, but you could only get a bed if it was your first or you had complications."**

It was recognised at this time that in some places the supply of beds was unequal to the demand, so in the 1950s the number of hospital beds increased so that the target set in 1959 by the Cranbrook Committee, of 'sufficient hospital beds to provide for a national average of 70% of all births to take place in hospital should be adequate to meet the needs of all women in whose case histories the balance of advantage appears to favour confinement in hospital', was reached by 1964. This was partly achieved by reducing the length of time a woman stayed in hospital after her baby was born. In 1951 the minimum recommended length of stay was 10 days. In 1955 the average stay was 12.1 days for a consultant bed and 11.1 for GP bed. By 1968 these had dropped to 8 and 6.8 respectively; this was because the birth rate had increased by 18 per cent while the number of beds had only grown by 15 per cent.

As the trend towards hospital birth increased, the numbers of hospital midwives swelled at the expense of the community midwives. By the late 1950s maternity homes became known as 'isolated GP units', although most deliveries there were done by midwives. These small units with approximately 12-15 beds were often much appreciated by their clients, but the British Perinatal Mortality Survey of 1958 expressed concern that such places lacked a resident medical officer and that anaesthetic facilities were limited. Since that time policy has favoured the creation of larger consultant units, often taking their mothers from a wide catchment area.

By 1970, when the Peel Report came out, only 12.4 per cent of babies were being born at home. It recommended that 'sufficient facilities should be provided to allow for 100 per cent hospital delivery. The greater safety of hospital confinement for mother and child justifies this objective.' As the numbers of hospital births grew there was a consequent drop in the numbers of midwives and doctors with experience of home birth who felt confident about conducting home confinements. Confidence has continued to be eroded and it is now quite usual for a midwife or doctor to qualify without having seen a home birth, let alone delivered a baby there.

In the 1970s the birth rate dropped, which resulted in an excess of maternity beds. This provided an opportunity for phasing out the small GP units that were not situated close to consultant units, so that the percentage of babies delivered in them fell to 5.7 per cent by 1978.

In 1980 the number of babies delivered at home was down to 1.2 per cent. It was in this year that the Social Services Committee recommended that 'an increasing number of mothers be delivered in large units; selection of patients is improved for small consultant units and isolated GP units and that *home delivery is phased out further* [author's emphasis]'. The figures show that the 1980s proved the low spot for home birth – the numbers dropped below 1 per cent and this includes the figures for babies whose mothers were booked to deliver in hospital but who, for one reason or another, delivered at home.

In 1993 the Winterton report was published. Nicholas Winterton, Chairman of the Health Select Committee, took care to listen to consumers[6] and found out what they needed from maternity services. His report stated that 'on the basis of what we have found this committee must draw the conclusion that the policy of encouraging all women to give birth in hospital cannot be justified on the grounds of safety'. The following year, the Changing Childbirth document[7] recommended that women should have more choice when deciding their place of birth and that more options should be available to them. The National Service Framework for Children, Young People and Maternity Services[8] in 2004 recommended active promotion of maternity care and that health care providers should develop midwife-led and home birth services to meet the needs of local populations. Today the latest figures for England and Wales (2004) show that the numbers of babies being born at home are growing – while still low at 2.4 per cent of all births, this is an increase of 7 per cent on the previous year. It is still no reflection of the numbers that would have been born at home had their mothers truly had a choice over where to give birth.

3 why women want their babies at home

"Why on earth do they ask where you want to have your baby when what they mean is – which hospital?"

For most of the world's women such a question doesn't arise – home is where you have babies unless major complications arise. However in the United Kingdom and the rest of the developed world (in some places, such as certain parts of the United States, home births are actually illegal) a woman wanting to have her baby at home may be expected to justify herself not only to her medical attendants but also perhaps to her partner, family and friends.

Of course there is no need to justify your decision, but it can help to analyse the reasons that are often cited for making a choice that is contrary to accepted practice today. They range from the purely pro-home to the actively anti-hospital.

One of the most often quoted reasons is the entirely justified one that the labour will be more relaxed and less stressful if it takes place at home, rather than moving at some point into the alien surroundings of a hospital. Unless you work in the hospital it is unlikely that you can feel really at home there, no matter how homely it is made to look. No one would deny that making hospitals less clinical in appearance is not a welcome change for those women who choose to have their babies in them, but they can never rival one's own home.

Clearly the degree of tension that going into hospital induces depends on the individual. Extroverts may feel it makes no difference, or merely be relieved to be in 'safe' hands. However, making a decision about leaving your familiar home and the freedom to do exactly as you please, and exchanging it for the bright lights and unfamiliar sights, sounds and smells of a busy hospital maternity unit must affect even the most outgoing to some extent. Animal studies show that interruption to some animals' labours can postpone labour or increase the rate of complications and perinatal mortality.[9] For those of us who are very private, entering a hospital can slow down or stop labour, to the point where it will require artificial stimulation to enable it to continue. The widespread use of pethidine in hospital is due to a need to relieve the tension caused by the paradox of needing to be relaxed in order to give birth while in strange and public surroundings in which privacy is negligible. This drug, which is rarely required at home, works more to relax the muscles than to relieve pain, although as tension increases awareness of pain it has a dual effect. Some women describe their feelings:

> "I'm the sort of person that can bear pain better than embarrassment and I warmed to the idea of giving birth in my own surroundings, in privacy, with just help from my husband and one or two midwives."

> "I felt I would be more comfortable and relaxed at home and more able to sleep."

> "We decided to have our baby at home because we knew it was the place where I would feel most relaxed. . . . The idea of our cosy, familiar bedroom as a birthplace appealed to us very much."

> "I came to my decision because I felt that I would be more relaxed in my own surroundings, whereas in hospital I knew I would be tense, apprehensive and worried that the whole process would be taken out of my hands."

> "Although I had worked at the hospital [as a midwife], seeing the labour ward as a pregnant woman made me frightened and uneasy. It seemed so clinical with equipment available for every kind of intervention possible; I had already decided I wanted minimum intervention."

It is not surprising that men as well as women find giving birth in a public place among people they do not know inhibiting. Conception is customarily an intimate affair, conducted away from others, generally at home or somewhere free from fear of interruption. Powerful social pressures mean that couples often suppress their intuitive feeling that birth should take place in similar conditions of privacy and security. As a result they bravely submit to hospital birth and relinquish their control of the situation. This, together with the unnecessary and routine use of medical intervention in the natural process of birth, are two of the more frequently stated reasons for rejecting birth in hospital.

For many adult independent women, pregnant for the first time, their treatment antenatally comes as a great shock. They complain bitterly of being expected to wait long hours for routine tests, of never seeing the same person twice, of being unable to establish a relationship with someone who will be present at the birth, but most of all as being regarded as stupid – "**I think they think you leave your brain at the door when you come in.**" They are disbelieved about the date of conception, not credited with feeling as they do, 'reassured' instead of listened to, patronised by doctors younger than themselves and generally told not to worry about things as they will be taken care of for them. For many, all this grates but they are prepared to tolerate it for the sake of the baby who is thought to benefit from this type of care. Others, although initially undecided about the place of birth, realise that similar attitudes may prevail during labour unless they take themselves out of the system.

"**I dreaded the hospital visits, and if I'd had any doubts about having my baby at home those visits certainly dispelled them.**"

"**When I started having children I assumed that the very best I could do for myself and my babies was to do as I was told. I trusted the professionals, believing them all to be wise and caring experts with a profound understanding of, and respect for, pregnancy, birth and motherhood. I was an 'easy patient', but bit by bit this touching faith was chipped away until, by halfway through my third pregnancy, I had become well and truly terrified of having another baby in hospital.**"

"**I felt strongly the need to be at home and in control of the situation.**"

Of course there are sympathetic and kindly midwives and doctors who will agree to be led by the parents', especially the mothers', wishes: but sadly, there are many more who, for reasons of training and their place in the hierarchy as well as for those of personal convenience and emotional comfort, will not listen to the mother. It is on these occasions – for example when restrictive or invasive monitoring of the fetal heart is insisted upon (despite many studies showing its lack of benefit and potential harm), when labour or its second stage is only 'allowed' to last a limited length of time without intervention, when pain relief is pressed upon the mother, when her requests are ignored because they do not comply with hospital policy, or treated with ill-disguised contempt – that women know they would be far happier had they stayed at home. However, such is the power of the propaganda that they may not even admit it to themselves. It is often these women who suffer not only at the time of birth but also after it. Loss of control in giving birth is a strong predisposing factor in subsequent postnatal depression, blighting the early period of motherhood and affecting the relationship with her new baby. (One study discovered a rate of postnatal depression of 60 per cent in mothers who had been delivered in hospital, compared with 16 per cent in women delivered at home.)

Tragically, previous bad hospital experiences often motivate women to have subsequent babies at home.

"My third baby was born at home after two hospital labours that I had no wish to repeat. On both occasions I was given drugs I'd rather not have had and both labours were spent immobile on the delivery table from two and a half centimetres onwards, resulting in more disorientation for me."

"I had a strap placed round my middle to monitor my contractions. Without consulting me the nameless doctor placed a wire up my vagina to monitor the fetal heart. I meekly protested, to which he replied 'Why not?' I felt assaulted and undermined by his attitude as more wire straps and belts were placed around me, inside me and next to me, thus immobilising me to the bed. I lapsed further into deferential. My labour was to be artificially controlled throughout and I felt powerless to protest."

Having a baby at home gives control back to a woman. Not only are the professionals on alien territory, a very significant alteration in the balance of power, but in most cases nothing will be done to her routinely or against her wishes. She is in a far better position to listen to her instincts and do exactly as she wants. She will not be inhibited by her surroundings. She will not have to make a decision to cut herself off from her everyday life and leave for hospital, removing herself from all the commonplace distractions and comforts that might take her mind off any pain she may be feeling. (One Canadian study found women giving birth at home reported feeling far less pain than their counterparts in hospital.[10]) She can more easily decline electronic monitoring; in fact the most restricting or invasive types, the cardiotocograph belt monitor and fetal scalp electrode, used for monitoring a baby in the absence of a midwife, are not yet available at home.

A woman at home will be able to labour slowly, there being no easy access to pharmacological methods of accelerating labour. In fact intervention is likely only to be used when there is a true indication as it generally involves a transfer to hospital, a situation which nearly everyone is keen to avoid. **"He was born at teatime, after a 15-hour labour (just as well we were at home, where no one could suggest spoiling it with Syntocinon)."**

In fact labour at home is often shorter than it would be in hospital. Not only can you be more relaxed about the whole process, comfortable in the knowledge that the midwife will come to you, but you can eat and drink freely and share your birth with anyone that you choose, including your children. Having friends with you can greatly increase the amount of physical and emotional support available to you; it has been shown to be superior to pethidine as a form of pain relief. Trusts vary in their policies as to who, apart from the father, you may have with you at a hospital birth. Moreover, although the father is allowed to be at the birth, he often feels redundant in hospital and can end up merely being used as a channel for conveying unwelcome information, as in 'Just tell your wife that we are going to do X, Mr Bloggs.' In accounts of birth at home, fathers are usually described as having plenty to do and in no way feeling superfluous.

"My husband was more at ease at home, with plenty of practical things to do ferrying children, feeding children and mid-

wives, providing gallons of tea, tending the fire."

"Mark's feet were hardly touching the ground – in between stroking my shoulders and back for just about every contraction, he was a great help. I requested (demanded) cardigan, arnica, hot water bottle, drink, flannel, cardigan off, sick bowl, door to bathroom to be closed, etc., etc."

Together you are on your territory and able to welcome your child into your home, a feeling which can be overwhelmingly 'right'.

"Having my baby at home kept birth in its normal place, alongside conception and pregnancy. Having to go away to hospital breaks up the experience dreadfully and its place in the normal sequence of family life is irretrievably lost. I felt whole, complete and happy – not disoriented and fragmented as in hospital."

Women often describe the anxiety and distress they feel at being parted from their husbands or partners right at the start of their life as a new family (see Jo's account of the first hours of her daughter's life on page 179). For many women it is the first time they have been parted from their partner and it comes at the very time when they most want the comfort of their company and need to share and discuss their feelings about the labour and their new baby.

"I also wanted to be *with* my family after the baby was born, to share this emotional and joyful event."

Fathers too experience a sense of anticlimax and loss when they are cast out on their own after sharing one of the most emotional moments of their lives. They are unable to get to know their babies immediately and miss most of their very earliest hours or days.

"Although he had been present at the birth of our daughters he had always felt somehow left out and inhibited and afterwards very deflated when he had to go home. In fact, we had always joked that it was him who had the 'baby blues' instead of me!"

Consideration of existing children is another reason given for having subsequent children at home. Women choose to do this rather than submit them to the double disruption caused by suddenly leaving them to go to hospital and then introducing them to the new baby there. Many mothers say this is their chief reason for home birth.

"I decided on a home birth for my third baby because I feel that a normal birth should be a part of family life. I saw no need for a hospital delivery in my case and I wanted my two older children, Hanna (six) and William (four), to view childbirth as a natural family event. They had been involved during the pregnancy and I didn't want to be separated from them when they had to cope with gaining a new brother or sister. As it turned out things went perfectly and they accepted Alexander into the family without any fuss."

"I thought they would benefit greatly by seeing their sister almost immediately after the birth."

"When I became pregnant for the second time, we decided we would like this baby to be born at home, mainly because we felt the atmosphere would be more relaxed, but also because I didn't want to be away from Sam."

"I felt a tremendous amount of resentment at having to leave my first child at home. I felt this baby has put me in hospital and it took me a long time to get to love him because I had been forced apart from my first."

Women whose babies have been born at home really do seem to find that it makes it easier for the other children to accept. A toddler's feelings at meeting a new brother or sister in hospital can only be guessed at. It must be daunting not only to find your mother in bed in totally strange surroundings in a room with a lot of other women, but also that the baby has her all to itself. It must be easier, if not necessarily more welcome, if the baby arrives without interrupting a child's routine. It is also far simpler for fathers if they do not have to take the whole family to a hospital for visiting twice a day, there to have to try and control the children while also giving attention to their wives and new baby.

Not only can brothers and sisters of home born babies see their new sibling just after the birth but, if you wish and it seems appropriate at the time, they can be present at the birth. This is simply not an option in hospital. Being at home means that, provided you have made prior arrangements to have them cared for at home or elsewhere if necessary, you can have them with you if it is what both you and they want at the time. As a mother of a seven-year-old daughter wrote, **"It meant a lot to me to have her there"**.

Some of the reasons for having a home birth are logistical. In remote areas the choice can be between having a baby at home or travelling up to 100 miles to a large hospital serving a wide area. In these cases obstetricians often like women to be admitted before their due date in order to await the birth, with obvious problems of separation from their families. Clearly there is a temptation to induce labour after a while. The national policy of closing small and often popular GP units in favour of centralised consultant units means that more women feel that home birth is the only reasonable alternative. Another factor related to NHS provision concerns the deterioration of services as a result of financial cuts. This applies especially to mothers hoping for a rest in hospital, or who prefer to be close to professionals used to caring for newborn babies for the first few days. Provision for hospital stay varies according to district, but can be as little as a maximum of 24 hours for a first birth. Some women feel that as the perceived benefits of a hospital stay are eroded, there is less to make having a baby there worthwhile. In fact even those mothers able to stay as long as they want generally discover that hospital, with its far-from-restful routines, busy wards and crying babies, is not the haven they had hoped for. It is true that the community midwife is not within shouting distance when you are at home, though she can easily be called in an emergency; but you have to assume responsibility for your baby at some point, and you may be more confident and less subject to conflicting advice if you do it right from birth. Babies, too, prefer not to move from the surroundings they become accustomed to after birth, and can be quite disturbed for a day or two after leaving hospital. In addition, one study of relative costs showed home birth to cost an average 30 per cent less than hospital.[11]

It may not be a deciding factor in the argument in favour of home birth, but birth in hospital does increase the risk of infection to both mother and baby: **"I observed that far from being a safe** place, a hospital was a fertile source of infection, which I could not reconcile with the birth of a vulnerable infant" (GP who had her baby at home). A survey organised by the National Childbirth Trust showed that in a comparison of women having home and hospital birth, 21.9 per cent of women in hospital contracted post-natal infection, against 4.9 per cent at home.[12] It may be that financial stringencies are responsible for the inadequate cleaning and removal of rubbish from the bathrooms and lavatories of maternity units, but the result is that infection rates are returning to pre-Victorian levels. Anecdotal evidence shows that women and babies are acquiring MRSA infections in hospital – scandalously, data regarding post-partum infection is not collated specifically.

The pressure of numbers in increasingly large hospital units must diminish the degree to which women are seen as individuals, despite efforts in some places to ensure continuity of care; it results in the 'conveyor belt' approach which is so disliked and yet difficult to avoid in hospitals where thousands of women give birth annually. Things are noticeably different if you elect to give birth at home. Not only will you be seen and remembered ante-natally (admittedly, not all the attention may be welcome), but your antenatal care may actually be in your home or at least at a neigbourhood surgery or clinic. When you are in labour you will be the centre of attention; the midwives will come to you and you will be treated as an individual. With luck they will have seen you throughout your pregnancy and you will have developed mutual trust and a good relationship. They will see you in your place as part of your family rather than the ninth one in labour that night. If you know them well, they will be aware of your hopes and wishes and be able to help you to achieve the birth you want. They will care for you until your baby is born, no matter how long it takes.

All these are appealing and convincing reasons for having a baby at home. However they will only appeal to those people who want and are prepared to take responsibility for themselves and their children. In deciding to have a baby at home you must recognise that you accept what will happen – both good and bad – and that in the unlikely event of an unavoidable disaster you will not seek to blame anyone else. Many people do wish to take on this responsibility, which after all is common to everyone once a baby leaves hospital, but unfortunately it is not always an option that is readily obtained.

"In Cornwall (or in this area of Cornwall anyway) they only allow 10 days over your due date before they want to induce mothers. I lied about the date of my last period. I added seven days, which proved to be just enough since I had the baby on the very day that they thought I was 10 days over (actually 17) and had made an appointment at the local maternity unit later that day. At just such an appointment in my first pregnancy the consultant had given me a cervical sweep which started me off later that day and resulted in an erratic and lengthy labour which I am sure was unnecessary.

"Following a hospital birth with my first baby which did not suit me at all, I set out in my second pregnancy to have a home birth. I would in fact have liked a home birth with my first baby but had been quickly discouraged at the outset by all the medical staff I came into contact with through the antenatal clinics, etc. I had been fortunate enough to meet Ann Garner, a very experienced midwife who was wholeheartedly in favour of home births whenever possible. Unfortunately she lived in Sheffield, which was much too far away for me to come under her care, but at least I had the opportunity to talk to her in depth about home births and get her reactions regarding my particular circumstances, i.e. that I was living in the country, many miles from the nearest hospital. She assured me that in my case she would not be concerned and if she worked in my area would happily deliver my baby at home.

"I knew in advance that the GPs at my surgery were not in favour of home births and was therefore pleasantly surprised when the midwife seemed very helpful and said that she would talk to her superiors about my request for a home birth and would try to find a doctor who would agree to cover it. However, at my next antenatal visit all my hopes became dashed when the midwife told me that her superior was totally against it because of the length of time that it would take an emergency flying squad to reach me and the fact that they could not find a doctor to cover me for a home birth. I confess to becoming tearful, as it seemed that they were saying I couldn't have a home birth. A normally strong, resilient type of person, I fought back the tears as I tried to tell them why I was so upset; that I felt I would have an easier birth at home because I would be happier and more relaxed in my own environment. It was not something I had thought of on a whim but something I had always believed in, even before contemplating a family. It was suggested that I went home and talked to my husband about it.

"My husband and I had, of course, already talked about it in depth and I wouldn't have liked a home birth if he had not agreed that, provided all was well, home was the best place to have our baby. Our feelings had not changed, the horror stories of possible consequences had not scared us into opting for a hospital, but it seemed hopeless as I was meeting brick walls at every turn. I hate having to admit that at around 30 weeks pregnant I felt vulnerable and didn't know whether I could carry on fighting the system. At one stage I even wondered if it would be easier just to give in and have the baby in hospital to save myself the anxiety I was having to cope with.

"At my next visit to the clinic I said that I still wanted to have the baby at home. Since no doctor would agree to cover, I accepted that I would have to rely on the midwife. They realised that I was not going to change my mind and from then on the midwife was very supportive and I think actually looked forward to delivering my baby at home.

"The necessary preparations were made and I was, after all, to have my baby at home. Remembering Ann Garner's suggestion, I spent about two hours of my labour in the bath – this proved to be excellent advice as it helped to make the contractions very easy to cope with. To give birth I adopted the squatting position and with three good pushes our baby was born. It really was very easy and I didn't feel like I had had a baby at all as I felt so good. It was truly wonderful and I was on cloud nine for weeks. It had been well worth the fight to have my baby at home – a decision I shall never regret."

"The unhappy experience of the birth of my first child convinced me that I wanted a home delivery next time round. It took place in a hospital that supposedly allowed gentle births, but I found the midwife and doctor who attended me to be unsympathetic. They wanted to accelerate the labour and tried to persuade me to take drugs to relieve the pain although the labour only lasted seven hours. They were cynical about natural birth, criticised my upright position during the second stage, and a nurse remarked 'It looks as if we have another over-protective mother' because I wanted to keep my baby close to me after he was born. I was told I must have an episiotomy 'just in case', and after I had been stitched up my baby was taken away for examination. He was brought back tightly wrapped in a sheet and, whereas he had been incredibly alert beforehand, now his eyes were tightly closed. I sat up cross-legged on the bed and began to unwrap him so I could look at him and cuddle him. Whether it was because I was sitting cross-legged(!) or because I wasn't doing just what I was told, I don't know, but a doctor came in and actually scolded me and asked 'Have you been taking drugs or something?' As I had spent my labour resisting the attempts by the hospital staff to persuade me to take drugs, I felt angry and humiliated. The whole thing was a battle and was made worse by the fact that I was alone there apart from the hospital staff. After this experience I realised that if birth is to take place in hospital it is essential to know exactly what you want in detail and to arm yourself beforehand with information to persuade unsympathetic staff that you know what you are doing.

"I felt good during my second pregnancy, I was attending yoga and childbirth classes with the emphasis on preparation for active birth.

"**Disappointed but undeterred** [by not getting a booking with an independent midwife] I went to my local clinic and the doctor there was enthusiastic about my having a home birth. It was a busy clinic and I saw many different midwives, although I would have preferred to get to know one midwife well and for her to deliver the baby.

"Two weeks before the baby was due I was resting after a shopping trip when I experienced a dull pain. When it recurred a few times I realised I was having contractions, so I began to record their frequency. They started about 12 noon, and about one o'clock my boyfriend Niall phoned the midwife. He was told to phone back because it was a Sunday and they couldn't contact a midwife who could come out at that moment. Niall's sister Mary arrived unexpectedly, which was great as she could help look after my two-year-old son. I was up and about, but whenever a contraction came, I stopped what I was doing.

"As the contractions became more intense I found it soothing and a lot of fun to sing loudly with my little boy Martin during a contraction. When I was ready to concentrate more fully, Mary took Martin for a walk and Niall phoned the midwife again. While he was doing that I was visited by the inquisitive four-year-old girl who lived in the upstairs flat. I tried to explain why I was squatting down and unable to talk to her properly during a contraction and I persuaded her to leave as soon as possible. It was so funny really as she was a very talkative and curious little girl, but I just couldn't cope with this at the time. Niall was told that a midwife had not yet been contacted and I would have to go into hospital if one could not be found.

"I decided to have a bath and the warm water was a great help in coping with the contractions, which by now were quite strong. Niall and Mary took turns at rubbing my back, which felt great; Martin had been taken to friends for a while. At around three o'clock I began to feel cold and a bit sleepy, the contractions had eased off a bit and I realised I was in transition. Luckily soon after a midwife did arrive, so I asked her to rub my back whilst Niall and Mary made preparations for the birth and she did this willingly. As our bed was on the floor level the midwife asked for something higher, so a single bed was put in the lounge where there was a fire. I then experienced a wonderful urge to push. During my first labour I did not experience this urge because I was not ready but had been instructed to push hard because the doctor wanted me to, which was unpleasant; by contrast this pushing urge felt so good. I was helped on to the single bed and started to push. The midwife had not even opened her bag yet and asked me to hold on until she got her instruments ready, but I couldn't; in fact no one had even remembered to close the curtains.

"The head was there and it was so exciting, then the midwife began to guide me, telling me when to push. I was most impressed by her skilful instructions – 'Push now', 'Just a little', 'Stop', 'Pant'. Danny was born without the slightest tear and I realised how much I had missed out in my first birth experience, when I was given a 'routine' episiotomy. Danny was probably two weeks early in actuality as well as by dates as he was covered with quite a lot of vernix. Everyone felt wonderful and high, including the midwife, who had never attended a home birth before and enjoyed it very much. The third stage was over quickly; the midwife had slipped in the ergometrine injection without asking as she was trained to do, and it was not something I was very aware about then, although now I would prefer not to have it. I had a bath while my bed was made up and the midwife bathed little Danny. I was too excited to sleep, so later on when the midwife called I was actually in the kitchen preparing a simple meal, while the baby slept. I felt fit and well, which I am sure owed a lot to the yoga preparation classes.

"The labour lasted less than four hours and I feel that because I was at home I wasn't inhibited by the stresses involved in leaving my home, meeting strangers and being in a hospital and so the labour went quickly and easily. I am delighted that I could have this experience and appreciated it all the more as my first labour and birth did not go well. My next three children were planned as home deliveries but had to be born in hospital as they were premature."

Catherine Morgan

"This is my third baby. I had two smooth labours, with no complications, and felt that this labour was sure to be straightforward in so far as one can be sure of anything in childbirth.

"I dislike hospitals and being subject to regulations and unwritten rules. When Cecily was born we only spent 25 minutes in hospital before she appeared. Christine [the midwife] said afterwards that if she had been able to come to us at home, as arranged by the domino scheme, Cecily would have been born there, as she wouldn't have wanted to move me in advanced labour. I remember thinking then that it was a pity it hadn't turned out like that, and that next time.... As Cecily and I came home eight hours after delivery, it didn't really seem worth the journey into hospital.

"Emotionally, I wanted to have this baby at home because I wanted him or her to be born in my own little nest with the rest of the family around. I wanted Adam and Cecily to meet the new member of the family without the strain of visiting in hospital or being separated even for a short amount of time. I wanted to be cared for by those I chose to look after me and whom I had invited into my home, rather than be subject to whoever happens to be on duty at the time – of course this might not have worked out, but was probably the biggest reason for my having chosen to have my baby at home.

"By knowing the midwives who were likely to deliver the baby and by choosing to have him or her at home, I felt I had done my best to ensure that there would be no unnecessary interference with the natural progression of labour. This meant that I felt confident and secure about the labour and as much in control of what happens as I wanted to be.

"I wanted the baby in with us, after the birth, in our bed, in our room, in our house – where he or she belonged. I had enjoyed organising the house, getting things right for the birth, the way we wanted them to be, rather than the best that could be managed in our understaffed, underfunded hospital which has to work to the rules.

"I felt excited and anticipatory about the birth, and much more relaxed about it than the previous two. Possibly it was just because it was my third and I knew a lot more about the mechanical side, but I think it had a lot more to do with knowing that I wouldn't have to go to hospital. I also felt happier that if I had to get Tony home from work, he only had to get here, and didn't then have to take me on to hospital.

"In the event, Isabel's birth was just what I wanted and expected. I gave it more thought beforehand than if I had been giving birth in hospital because I knew I had far more control over what would happen. With a hospital birth you can say what you want but there is no guarantee that you will get it.

"I had a feeling that I was doing it all myself, although that is partly due to Christine, my midwife, who is so good at letting you feel like that. Having people that I knew around me was the most helpful thing.

"I was surprised at how uninhibited I was at home. I would have thought that I would be less inhibited in impersonal hospital surroundings, and more concerned about making a noise at home and disturbing the neighbours. However, making a noise helped and I wasn't worried about doing it. I was also surprised that I didn't tear (Isabel weighed 9 lb 8 oz) and I think that was a result of being so relaxed at home.

"I especially enjoyed having my children and my parents there straightaway. It was lovely to be in my own setting and very calming to get back into our own bed. We managed to get a couple of hours sleep that night, which I'm sure I would not have done in hospital, and every bit of sleep helps at that stage."

Liz Crawley

4   safety

Perhaps the most persistent and striking feature of the debate about where to be born however, is the way policy has been formed with very little reference to the evidence.

Where To Be Born

It seems hard to credit that the policy of nearly 100 per cent hospital births can have been so relentlessly pursued on the basis of an assumption rather than carefully collected statistics, but this is the case. Unfortunately for women wanting to give birth at home, a drop in the perinatal mortality rate (the number of stillbirths and babies dying in the first week of life) coincided with the increase in hospital deliveries. This was regarded as sufficient evidence to continue to endorse the trend, regardless of expense, although, as it will be seen, it is probable that the perinatal mortality rate would have dropped still further had the policy favouring hospital birth not been encouraged.

That the assumption has been challenged is largely due to the valiant efforts of Marjorie Tew, to whom a great debt is owed by those women who want evidence to support their belief that birth at home is best for themselves and their babies. Mrs Tew was a research statistician in the Department of Orthopaedic Surgery at Nottingham Medical School. She first became interested in the issue when she set her students an exercise to prove the truth that birth was safest in hospital, and found with incredulity that the case was not proven at all. From then on she worked tirelessly, coping not only with the reluctance of the authorities to part with the available statistics but also with the reluctance of the obstetricians and policymakers to accept them. Her findings included the following:

- There is some evidence, although not conclusive, that morbidity [disease or abnormality] is higher among mothers and babies cared for in an institutional setting. For some women the iatrogenic risk [that caused by the process of diagnosis or treatment] associated with institutional delivery may be greater than any benefit conferred, but this has yet to be proven.

• A majority of women who have experienced both home and hospital deliveries prefer to have their babies at home, although this may include a disproportionate number of women who have sought home delivery after a hospital delivery with which they were dissatisfied.

Of course most of this data is concerned with the measurable statistics of perinatal mortality and of course women would rather lose a beautiful birth experience than a baby. They would and do have their babies in hospital, subjugating their own desires, in the belief that they are giving their babies a better chance. The British evidence, together with studies from Holland, suggests that birth is safer at home, with fewer complications in pregnancy, delivery or the puerperium.[13] It looks as though by having a baby in hospital you are doing both the baby and yourself a disservice.

As stated before, obstetrical interventions have, until recently, been introduced without prospective, controlled trials; that is, allocating women into two groups before the intervention is performed and then using the intervention on only one group. As far as possible there should be no other difference, other than the particular intervention, so that the groups are matched for age, class, number of children and so on. Of course it is difficult to do this with something so individual as giving birth, where attitudes and relationships can so greatly affect the outcome, and it is largely impossible to do double-blind trials where neither doctor nor midwife knows what the mother is receiving, as is the case in well-organised drug trials. None the less it is important that no intervention should gain widespread acceptance without its benefits being clearly proven first.

Fortunately this need has now been recognised. For example, consumer groups such as the Association for Improvements in the Maternity Services (AIMS) and the National Childbirth Trust (NCT) have welcomed the opportunity offered to assist in designing a trial to evaluate the benefits, risks and long-term effects of chorionic villus sampling (an early test for abnormality which involves removing a small piece of placental tissue via the vagina).

However, this is a new development; most evaluations of interventions are retrospective and only performed after the techniques have been in use for some time. Many studies have been carried out, on everything from the use of salt as an antiseptic in postnatal bathwater to the benefits of continuous monitoring and the value of inducing overdue babies. Disturbingly, the results frequently show that the benefits of such interventions, which frequently cause great distress to mother and baby, not only are non-existent but are actually harmful. Worse, they continue to be used even in the face of the evidence of their worthlessness.

It is worth briefly examining these interventions and the evidence that refutes them in order to be persuaded of the truth of Marjorie Tew's conclusions.

ULTRASOUND

This is used routinely on pregnant women in the UK, allegedly to estimate fetal age (this being held to be more reliable than a woman's recollection of the dates of her period and the length of her cycle or even her idea about the date of conception), to detect abnormality and babies at risk from retarded intrauterine growth. It is also used in procedures such as amniocentesis and chorionic villus sampling. The technique was introduced without proper evaluation and it is still too early to be certain that it does not have lasting side-effects. The Department of Health has recommended that it is not used routinely, and it is used much less extensively in the United States where obstetricians seem more aware of the theoretical risk in its use.[14] More information about ultrasound is available on the AIMS website, **www.aims.org.uk.**

Although ultrasound is popular with some mothers, it can be responsible for lasting anxiety in mothers if minor abnormalities are detected in pregnancy. The distress that this can cause, even when the problem turns out to be nonexistent at birth, should not be underestimated. This might be considered justifiable if in all other respects ultrasound assessments were accurate. Unfortunately, there is evidence to show that not only are they inaccurate in detecting small-for-dates babies (those who have not grown well in the uterus) but that inducing labour in those women who are thought to have babies in this category can result in the birth of normally-growing but premature babies; further-more, the induction of labour does not benefit babies that are gen-uinely growth retarded. Another study showed that measuring the mother's abdomen with a tape-measure proved a better predictor of poor fetal growth than a series of three and sometimes four scans in pregnancy.[15]

The degree of success in accurately determining the presence or absence of fetal abnormality is dependent upon the skill and expe-rience of the operator, and is far from 100 per cent, even in centres of excellence. As case histories included in this book demonstrate, it is not infallible either way. As Hazel says in her birth story, there may be no point in having one if, in the event of a major abnormal-ity being detected, you would not contemplate termination any-way (see page 209).

INDUCTION

The percentage of induced labours is falling but it is still largely regarded as necessary to induce labours at any time from full-term to (more commonly) 10-12 days over the due date, to protect babies from the risk of death due to post-maturity. The length of time 'allowed' depends on the policy of the consultant. This is in spite of the fact that studies show that the baby is at no greater risk if the pregnancy continues up to 44 weeks, if monitored.[16]

A prospective study of women booked for home birth and a control group booked for hospital birth found twice as many labours in the hospital group were induced.[17] The hazards of induced labour have been well documented by Sally Inch in her book *Birthrights*: they include an increased risk of infection in mother and baby; an increased likelihood of epidural, forceps and Caesarean section; postpartum haemorrhage has been shown to occur nearly twice as frequently; the baby is more likely to be asphyxiated and require special care; it is more likely to become jaundiced and to be affected by the greater use of pharmacologi-cal pain relief by its mother. All these are physiological hazards; they do not include the lasting psychological damage done to women who feel an enduring sense of loss and failure at not hav-ing gone into labour spontaneously.

CONTINUOUS FETAL MONITORING

This is one of the most discredited types of intervention. The Royal College of Obstetricians and Gynaecologists recommendations from the 26th RCOG Study Group: Intrapartum Fetal Surveillance now recognises that continuous fetal monitoring is not beneficial in normal labour. Eight studies, covering vast numbers of women (35,000 in one American trial), have shown that continuous fetal monitoring does not improve the outcome for the baby and may actually harm it.[18] Caesarean section and forceps rates (33 per cent in one case) are increased for those women undergoing continuous fetal monitoring because distress is detected and acted upon more frequently, but the babies' chances of survival were not improved by these operative deliveries. This is perhaps because fetal heart rate monitoring is picking up indications of distress that are normal in labour but which were previously undetected because less sophisticated forms of monitoring made it difficult to hear the fetal heart during a contraction. This can explain why babies delivered operatively because of 'fetal distress' often show no signs of being distressed, i.e. do not have a lowered Apgar score at birth (see page 84).

The risks to the baby include infection, abscess and the misplacing of the scalp electrode. The risks to the mother, besides that of unnecessary operative delivery, also include infection, as well as the increase in anxiety levels, pain of insertion, restriction of movement, inhibition of labour, etc. − things which may be ignored in an assessment of the value of such monitoring.[19] And indeed, the NICE draft guidelines (June 2006, page 409) state that 'there is high level evidence that women who had routine admission CTGs were more likely to have interventions during labour, although there were no statistical differences in neonatal outcomes'.

ROUTINE CAESAREAN SECTION FOR BREECH BABIES

Again, depending on the consultant, a baby in the breech position is regarded as a candidate for automatic Caesarean section.[20] These babies, previously delivered at home by midwives, are now regarded as constituting major obstetric problems in many hospitals, and many women with babies in the breech position are simply not allowed to deliver them vaginally.[21] A review of all the literature by two American authors (Myers and Gleichen) concludes that routine Caesarean section for breech presentation is unnecessary and costly.[22] Moreover a retrospective casenote review of births in a Liverpool hospital found that breech presentations discovered in labour were more likely to deliver vaginally than those that had been detected and given a trial of labour. The babies showed no sign of suffering as a consequence.[23]

EPIDURAL

Although this is not an intervention that is offered routinely, the use of epidurals and pethidine has been shown to be much higher amongst first-time mothers booked to deliver in consultant units than in those booked to deliver at home or in low-tech GP units with community midwives or GPs. The babies born in the GP unit or at home have been shown to be in better condition at birth, they had higher Apgar scores, and required less intubation (when a tube is inserted into the lungs to assist breathing) than babies who were born in the consultant unit.

Epidurals should only be administered by a trained anaesthetist and so are not available at home; pethidine is available at a home birth but is very rarely needed as the situation decreases a woman's awareness of pain. Other disadvantages of epidurals include: their failure to work either partially or totally; the risk of the needle puncturing the dura – resulting in a severe headache for several days; it affecting the nerve supply to your lungs so that you cannot breathe; a reduction in blood pressure leading to fetal distress; an increase in forceps deliveries; and long-term backache or, very rarely, paralysis.

Pethidine, which may be pushed by hospital staff, also has some well-documented side-effects. For example, it can have an adverse effect on the baby's breathing when given too close to the birth; this effect can be reversed by giving the baby an injection of naloxone at birth, although this is not entirely satisfactory because the effects of the antidote last for a shorter time than the effects of the pethidine. Some women also find that pethidine causes drowsiness, nausea, vomiting, and a feeling of being disassociated from the birth. Others report horrific hallucinations. Its strength is in acting as a relaxant to counter the tension and inhibition induced by attempting to give birth in surroundings in which the woman does not feel comfortable. A Danish study showed that four times more pethidine was needed in hospital compared with those giving birth in an alternative birth centre.[24]

WITHHOLDING FOOD AND DRINK IN LABOUR

This is no longer policy – women will be allowed a light diet – but they may not get it. Policy is not always translated into practice. The latest NICE recommendations (consultation draft document June 2006) are that 'women may take a light diet during labour . . . and that women should be encouraged to drink during labour and be informed that isotonic sports drinks are more beneficial than water.' However 'high-risk' women are still not permitted anything to eat or drink.

It is still useful to include the information about the effects of such a policy here, though not only as an example of the way in which interfering with the normal course of labour can have extremely serious consequences, and to show how misguided blanket policies can be; but also to demonstrate the value of maintaining your strength in labour.

Another common practice is that of not permitting women to eat and drink in labour, 'just in case they need a Caesarean'. This is because of the fear that in the eventuality of a woman requiring a general anaesthetic for an emergency Caesarean section, she might vomit food or drink and inhale the vomit, causing a lethal failure of the lungs. Research has shown, though, that not only is it extremely unlikely that aspiration will take place if she is allowed to eat and drink as she wishes in labour, but the contents of a so-called empty stomach are in fact filled with gastric acids which are very caustic and would cause more harm to the lungs if inhaled than partially digested food.

There were no cases of inhalation of vomit amongst 20,000 births in N. Central Bronx hospital when the mothers were allowed to eat and drink freely, but when they instituted a trial of starvation in labour for a six month period, it increased the rate of instrumental delivery by 35 per cent, of Caesarean section by 38 per cent, decreased the likelihood of a vaginal delivery after a previous Caesarean section by 37 per cent, and increased the need for babies to receive intensive care by 69 per cent.[25] Moreover, the common practice of combining starvation with oral antacids caus-es greater damage to be done to the lungs in the event of aspira-tion than if the stomach held clear fluid.

Starvation is recognised as causing problems other than those listed above. Ketonuria, the presence of ketones in the urine of the labouring woman (which indicates the body is deriving its energy directly from body fat), was conventionally treated by putting the woman on a drip containing glucose solution in water. (Because ketosis also slows the process of labour it may now be treated by accelerating labour artificially.) Two papers in the June 1988 volume of *Birth* suggest that, not surprisingly, this causes problems of its own. Not only do they suggest that some ketosis is normal in labour, and therefore should not be treated except by allowing the woman to eat and drink lightly, but they list the considerable dis-advantages of a glucose drip. These include: infection; the risk of maternal and fetal hyperglycaemia (too much sugar), which can lead to fetal hyperinsulinism (too much insulin), neonatal hypogly-caemia (too little sugar) and neonatal jaundice. This is on top of the discomfort of the drip, the restriction of movement and the endorsement of the women's status as a patient rather than a mother. The authors suggest that as women at full-term are carrying an extra 2 litres of water, it is unlikely that she will become dehy-drated in any way; they feel that 'partial dehydration and moderate ketosis may well be a normal and even beneficial part of labour and may be essential in protecting the fetal brain from hypoxic damage'.

GROUP B STREPTOCOCCUS (GBS)

Group B streptococci are a normal inhabitant of the body. Prophylactic treatment of women to prevent the small chance of their passing it to their babies is currently causing a lot of difficul-ty in the UK. A small number of babies (1 in 1,000) develops an infec-tion after birth as a result of becoming colonised by GBS, general-ly as a result of acquiring it from their mothers following the rup-ture of membranes before or during birth, although 20 per cent get the infection after the second day of life when it is presumed to have been acquired in other ways. Seven hundred babies born in the UK each year are affected and sadly 10 per cent of them die as a result.

The trouble is caused by the fact that the bacteria is a normal constituent of the bodies of a third of the population and 25 per cent of women carry it in their vaginas without it causing any problem or symptom. Many, many babies have been born (and still are) to women carrying the bacteria, without anyone being the wiser. A vaginal swab taken around 37 weeks of pregnancy may show (the NHS test has a 50% false negative rate) whether a woman carries Strep B in her vagina. Should this be the case, she will be offered intravenous antibiotics in labour for a minimum of four hours. Should this not be possible, her baby will be given antibiotics after birth. Due to the false negative testing rate, it has been suggested that even those with negative tests should have intravenous antibiotics during labour (in fact there is a more accurate test – ECM – which is only available privately). In theory every labouring woman should be given intravenous antibiotics which are effective in reducing infection rates from 1 in 300 babies of women known to have vaginal GBS, to 1 in 6,000.

Strep B information can be alarming and is used to insist on women giving birth in hospital. Intravenous antibiotics can be given at home, although it is unlikely to be part of most people's home birth dream, and may not be easy to arrange. You may want to consider it if you have already had a baby with Strep B, if your membranes have been ruptured for over 24 hours (although see the NICE guidelines on PROM), if your temperature is above 37.8 degrees Centigrade in labour, or if GBS has been detected in your urine during pregnancy (this should have been treated with antibiotics at the time).

It is not known why just one of those 300 babies is susceptible when 299 are not.

If you are shown to carry Strep B vaginally, it might be best to work on improving your health and that of your baby by ensuring that you have a good diet, eating lots of green leafy vegetables and plenty of garlic to boost your immunity.

If you have been shown to grow GBS, it is still possible to have a water birth; it is also possible to treat it with intramuscular (IM) antibiotic injections weekly between 36-40 weeks of pregnancy. There must be some concern about taking antibiotics prophylactically however – even more about giving them to newborn babies when not required. Oral antibiotics in pregnancy do not appear to be effective in preventing GBS in babies. More information is available from **www.gbss.org.uk**.

Signs of illness in very young babies include:

- grunting
- poor feeding
- lethargy
- irritability
- high/low temperature
- high/low heart rate
- high/low breathing rate
- unusual cry
- tense, bulging soft spot (fontanelle)
- stiffness or tension in moving
- pale or blotchy skin
- floppiness
- staring expression

Any of these are indications to seek medical help immediately. Better safe than sorry.

Conclusion

All these examples suggest that, as many women believe intuitively, imposing man-made interventions on the normal physiological process of labour, in the absence of strong and undeniable indications, is at best misguided and at worst wilful ignorance. It is clear that giving birth in the comfort and security of your own home, with the very minimum of interference, is likely to produce the best outcome for you and the baby – and this is only in the crude terms of measurable physical condition. It is difficult to quantify the difference in terms of how a woman feels about herself, about her achievement in giving birth rather than being delivered and about her lifelong relationship with her baby.

This is not to claim that intervention is never necessary or on occasion life-saving; just to demonstrate that it is not normally required and that abnormal cases would be far fewer without its routine application. But there is no point in amassing the available evidence if the person you hope to persuade is not open to reason. Sadly, as the examples in Chapter 6 show, those who might be expected to pay the closest attention to scientific evidence – obstetricians, doctors and midwives – frequently show the least regard for the facts.

5 deciding to have your baby at home

"I am beginning to feel very isolated over this matter and am almost afraid to approach anyone for fear of another browbeating over how stupid I am being. My husband respects my wishes, but is constantly accosted by people who 'wouldn't let my wife do it' and tell him tales of death, gloom and gore . . ."

Given that to choose to have a baby at home is to swim against the tide of current opinion, when should you make the decision and what reaction, other than medical, will you get? Can it be regarded as primarily your decision or will you be deterred if your partner is not in favour?

A surprising percentage of women make the choice even before becoming pregnant for the first time. At the other extreme there are those who beg an independent midwife to book them for home birth only when they are threatened with induction because their baby is overdue. You may feel happier if you get your home booking established right from the start; this certainly has the advantage of providing an opportunity to get to know the community midwives and it makes the need for provision clear to those responsible for planning it. Some people think that this increases your chances of giving birth at home. It also means that you can avoid all the hospital visits.

On the other hand you may opt for a late booking, either because you cannot really focus on the birth until it is only a few weeks away, or because you do not really appreciate what giving birth in hospital will be like until you have been on your hospital tour, or perhaps because you feel that it is not worth battling with until the birth is imminent. If for any reason you do feel that you want a last-minute change of booking, do not be deterred by a fear of upsetting people. There may not be any enthusiasm for it, but can be done right up until the baby is born. True, you may not get to know the midwife, but this is what you would expect if you were delivering in hospital anyway. People can and do book for home delivery on the community at 40 weeks and later.

You may anticipate opposition from some doctors and mid-wives, but what about your family and friends? Often a partner, subject to the same propaganda as women are about place of birth, will be apprehensive. He may be unable to appreciate quite why it is so important to you, or may not share your confidence in your ability to give birth unaided. He may feel that you and the baby are both his responsibility and that the question of whether home birth is putting either of you at risk is ultimately his to answer. He may believe that hospital is the safest place, may perhaps feel more empathy with technology than you do, or not know any fathers whose children have been born at home. Iain's story on page 47 illustrates many of these feelings. In most cases reluctant partners can be persuaded to agree by being given the facts to read and by taking the opportunity to speak to other fathers who have been through it themselves. Your nearest home birth support group (details from **www.homebirth.org.uk**) can be invaluable for putting men in touch with each other and providing an opportunity to hear first-hand from fathers what the experience was like for them. You can point out that he will have a real part to play at the birth rather than feeling redundant, as some men do in hospital. If you already have children it can be a great boon not to have to take them into the hospital to meet the baby, where children are not always wel-come and when it can be difficult to devote enough attention to you and the baby while keeping an eye on the other children. Often the father who has had reservations becomes an enthusiastic advo-cate once he has actually seen his baby born in his home.

Some fathers, however, will not agree, which poses a problem – should you shelve the idea, it being his baby too, or is your baby ultimately your responsibility as you are carrying it and will give birth to it, whether he is there or not? Only you can make this deci-sion. It will certainly be harder to do it if you do not have support within your own home, but it is not impossible. It may help if you can explore his fears, talking them out to the most extreme conclu-sion.

If the reaction you get from the rest of your family and your friends is negative too, you may need support from other women that you know to be in favour of home birth. Home birth can arouse violent emotions and you may be taken aback by the force of the feelings other people have about it. However, you may find unexpected support from older women who had their babies at home, some of whom find it hard to understand what all the fuss is about. Others may be ambivalent, feeling that home birth was fine for them but having an impression that hospital is necessary now. Your parents or your parents-in-law may feel uneasy, concerned for the baby as well as for you.

It can be upsetting to be undermined by those opposed to your ideas. This is made worse when you feel emotional and vulnerable because you are pregnant and are only doing what you think is best. It can seem that in choosing home birth you have set yourself up as a target for everyone to advise you of your folly, regardless of the fact that otherwise your emotional welfare would be treated with care.

For various reasons your peer group may be the most doubtful. This may be because they may have never questioned the belief that hospital is safer, they may know of no one else who has done it, or simply because it seems to be an unconventional and threatening stance. They can also be envious or resentful if they have felt misgivings about hospital birth but courageously had their babies there, feeling they had no other option. Common comments will be 'Aren't you brave' and 'What if something goes wrong?' If you feel like it you can give them the facts, although you may not want to be involved in endless debate. However, spreading awareness and clarifying the facts can make it easier for others to take the same option.

If it all becomes too much – and it can become isolating – you can claim to be going to the nearest hospital. And in the end it can be easier, if not ideal, to get a home birth by keeping your head down right until the end and then just refusing to go into hospital.

If you do find yourself feeling isolated about having a baby at home, contact anyone from one of the home birth support groups, who will understand how you feel and give you hope and encouragement. They will be happy to give you continued help throughout pregnancy and will provide a welcome opportunity to discuss any worries and anxieties you may have. This is especially valuable if you feel you are only grudgingly being allowed a home booking; in such a situation you may not feel able to discuss things freely with your doctor or midwives, although you should always mention anything that might have a bearing on your health or that of your baby. Other sources of help and support include the Association for Improvements in the Maternity Services, the Association of Radical Midwives, the Independent Midwives Association and the Midwives Information and Resource Service (see Useful Addresses).

"After having my first son in hospital, I was determined to have any subsequent babies at home. I had been unhappy with the interference and 'clinical' way in which I was treated during my first labour; the 'natural' birth I had envisaged gave way to strange faces, drips and total agony.

"When I became pregnant with my second son, I had absolutely no doubts in my mind regarding his birth place; I wanted to be at home, where I would be totally relaxed with my family. However, my GP (a young female doctor) was not prepared to offer me medical cover, and the same attitude against home births prevailed amongst all the doctors at my current practice. The consultant at the hospital had me in tears at my first visit, telling me what an 'irresponsible' decision I was making, and practically refusing there and then to have any-thing to do with me. He was totally against home births; not having had to deal with one for eight years, he saw it as a step backwards.

"From these initial reactions I began to understand why women allow themselves to be led into believing that hospital births are 'safer'. If I had not been so stubborn and determined I may well have given into the system – I had people from all directions shaking their heads and looking aghast at the mere mention of home births; and at a time when one is feeling par-ticularly vulnerable and emotional it is not easy to stand up to all the so-called experts.

"Finally I was given very helpful advice which was to write to the local Supervisor of Midwives, who is responsible for organ-ising maternity cover by midwives for all pregnant women in her district. I was also told a GP was not needed.

"I was assigned a midwife, who undertook all my antenatal care; this way I was able to get to know my midwife who would be present at my labour, and consequently my confidence in her and her continuous care throughout resulted in my totally relaxed state during labour.

"Together, Phyllis (my midwife) and I fought against the petty rules and prejudices, such as the fact that I was not allowed to attend any antenatal clinic but had to be seen separately and we even had to battle for my right to use clinic facilities. But it was nice to have someone on my side, and slowly we got our way.

"The labour went beautifully. I began having mild contractions at about 3.30 am on the Tuesday morning before Christmas, and immediately phoned Phyllis (who was up wrapping presents, unable to sleep!). By the time she got here the contractions were quite strong – Mark my husband and my sister Tracey were making me cups of tea and rubbing my back whilst I crouched in the lounge.

"Phyllis examined me in the bedroom and realised I was very close. We discussed whether she should phone for assistance, but both agreed it was unnecessary. I felt very calm and in control and had the utmost faith in my midwife.

"I have a large rocking chair in the bedroom in which I had planned to give birth, but when the time came I felt more comfortable being propped upon the bed.

"Joel was born at 5.50 am after a very joyous and happy labour. Unlike my first birth, I needed no stitches and Joel was put straight to the breast. He weighed a healthy 8 lb. I remember feeling so very proud of myself and my 'little team', because, despite all the odds against us from the start, we had done it.

"Hopefully Phyllis and I had paved the way for other mums wishing to have a home birth. In fact Phyllis has now informed me that she is undertaking the care of four women in the district who wish to have home births."

Karen Condon

"As my first baby was arriving into this world, almost as exhausted as I was, my immediate thought was 'Thank goodness I didn't have forceps: now I can have the next one at home'. No, I hadn't had a dreadful experience in hospital; I just knew that, for me, the place to have a baby was at home. In retrospect I even wish I'd had the courage to have the first one at home but, being a midwife myself, four years of indoctrination had nearly convinced me that the only place to have babies was in hospital.

"So I entered my second pregnancy, ten months later, knowing that I wanted to have the baby at home. I expected to meet a lot of opposition but my mind was set.

"Before I was pregnant, I broached the subject with my husband. He was not totally convinced, especially about the safety aspects, but felt that in view of my professional qualifications, he would respect my decision and stand by it.

"Booking a midwife was no problem as my ex-colleagues were more than happy (if not delighted) that I had chosen to have a home birth.

"The next hurdle to meet was my GP. I knew that he firmly opposed 'these silly women that want to have their babies at home'. I realised that I didn't have to have medical cover, but I preferred not to alienate my GP, especially as I have great respect for his professional capabilities. Much to my amazement, faced with a well-informed, determined patient asking for a home birth, he raised no objections.

"So the booking was confirmed, very easily as it happened. In fact, looking back on the months of pregnancy, the only opposition I ever encountered was from my peer group. They were most surprised that a midwife, of all people, was willing to risk having a baby at home.

"Without lapsing too much into superlatives, my labour and delivery went without a hitch. Looking back on four years of midwifery, I had never been present at such a perfect labour and delivery, and what was more it was my own. I was so relaxed and in tune with my body's needs. Admittedly it was a short labour and easy delivery, but my sister, who was looking after my 19-month-old son, commented afterwards that it was as if I had gone upstairs for a bath and the next thing she heard was a baby crying.

"At this point I have to express my eternal gratitude to a wonderful community midwife (and friend) who made it all possible.

"The best part, though, was the ensuing days. It was great to be in my own home; to have a lovely warm bath straight after the baby was born; to have a freshly cooked meal a few hours later (in hospital, after my first baby was born, they forgot to give me breakfast, so I had to wait eight hours for my first meal, and I was starving); to have cups of tea and coffee when I wanted them; generally to be able to eat, sleep, drink whenever I pleased. However good hospital is, it can never replace one's home comforts.

"So my third pregnancy was embarked upon with no doubts in anyone's mind. The baby would be born at home again. Even my GP didn't broach the subject of a hospital birth. The fact that my first home birth had been so a-problematic seemed to justify my choice for our third child.

"My husband by this stage had become totally convinced of the benefits. Having a home birth was so easy! No worrying about getting a labouring wife to hospital in time, no visiting problems, no babysitters needed for the children.

"One amusing sideline during my pregnancy was that I couldn't find any children's books which explained that babies could be born at home. My three-and-a-half year old and two year old were quite bewildered by the pictures of ambulances and hospitals in the 'new baby' books, as I kept telling them our baby would be born at home,

"Leaving aside the details of a rather long drawn-out labour and delivery, once again I look back on that day with immense pride and satisfaction. I laboured overnight, attended by my husband and midwife, who played endless board games. Eventually I delivered at 5 o'clock; the baby and I bathed together; the bedroom returned to its normal state; and then, as the midwives were leaving, our two children woke up. My husband and I brought them into our bedroom to 'discover' the new baby. After the excitement of exchanging presents, we dressed the children and all went down to the kitchen for breakfast. It was as if nothing had happened – except of course that the baby had mysteriously arrived overnight. No fuss, no bother – just very simple, just perfect."

Jenny O'Keefe

"It was early in my first pregnancy that I realised I wanted to give birth at home. My biggest problem in arranging the birth was that I didn't know where I would be living at the time my baby was due. My partner and I were living in a rented flat, from which we were about to move, when I found I was pregnant. The next flat we found was only for six months, so I knew I would have to move yet again before the baby was born. Knowing this, I sadly put the idea of a home birth out of my mind. I thought that maybe I could find the lesser of the evils in the right hospital. So I shopped around.

"I decided to book at a hospital which had a reputation for natural childbirth and letting women labour with as little medical intervention as possible. I went on a tour of the hospital, had a hundred questions answered, and felt quite confident that this hospital was almost as good as being at home.

"For the duration of my pregnancy, I was constantly reading about the process of labour and hospital procedures – basically anything about the subject I could get my hands on. The idea of a home birth still tugged at me, but as long as where we were to live was up in the air, I thought it best to prepare myself for a hospital birth.

"By the time my antenatal classes started it was about time for us to move again. I was then about seven weeks away from giving birth. The antenatal classes shook my faith in the hospital. I was getting conflicting information at the classes to that which I had been told at the hospital tour. It disturbed me to find, so close to delivery, that hospital policies and procedures that had influenced my decision on this particular hospital were not at all consistent with the information I had first received. I feared that, to give birth naturally there, I would have to fight for it all through labour; unless I was lucky to get a midwife who was willing to bend the policies.

"Finally at four weeks away from giving birth, my partner and I found a flat in Twickenham. We moved in on a Saturday and the following Monday I had a hospital antenatal check-up. I had begun to consider strongly a home birth again, since I then knew where I was going to be when the baby arrived. I was nervous to try for it, though, for fear of a possible fight to arrange it, as I didn't have much time left before the big event. But it was the hospital check-up on Monday that helped me make up my mind.

"Half of the medical gadgetry used to examine me didn't work and the doctor examining me wasn't shy to say that the whole hospital was falling apart. Then when it came to discussing some of my birth plans that I wanted recorded on my notes, the doctor became indignant. I had checked at the tour that all my birth plans aligned with their policies, so the doctor's reaction again accentuated the uncertainty of the hospital's reputation for natural birth and its attitudes towards permissiveness to a labouring woman's wishes.

"After a long heated discussion I left feeling very uneasy. The doctor had told me there was a 50/50 chance of getting the type of birth I wanted there. This was not something I wanted to hear less than a month away from delivery. If that wasn't enough, I was trying to get some information from the sister before I left and she was extremely rude and short with me. The whole hospital environment set me ill at ease.

"When my husband arrived home that evening he told me that he had taken the liberty of calling the clinic in our area that would book me a home birth. He said they were quite positive and would send a midwife in the middle of the week to discuss it.

"That evening, though, at 11.30 my waters broke. We then had a real dilemma. We decided to call the hospital for lack of a better idea. All my books advised me to call straight away if the waters go right at the beginning of labour. Our phone was not connected yet, since we had just been moved two days, so my husband and I walked down to the phone box at the top of our street. I kept telling him I wasn't going into hospital, because I knew they would try to convince him.

"Once he got through to the labour ward and explained that I was booked there and my waters had broken, they began trying to coerce him into bringing me into hospital. He made it clear that I wasn't going to go. He explained that we were in the process of planning a home birth, but the midwife wasn't due to visit and arrange it until the middle of the week. We hadn't expected the baby to arrive three and a half weeks early. He then asked if a community midwife could just come to our home to check me. To our surprise they agreed to our request.

"We returned home and waited. I ran through in my head just what I would say to the community midwife when she arrived. I couldn't be certain how agreeable she would be to what would seem to some as irrational behaviour.

"Once she arrived, I quickly began explaining how we had wanted a home birth; that our decision was an educated one as we knew all about birth and hospital procedures. And that, simply, I just wanted to get on with having my baby without the fear of being unnecessarily interfered with.

"Her reaction was a welcome contradiction to that which I had originally psyched myself up for. She understood why I wanted to stay in my own home and was quite happy to help me achieve the natural birth I had so diligently prepared for. She didn't think me irrational at all.

"I trusted her skill and judgement as a midwife and knew she would not have been so sympathetic to my desire to stay at home had there been any abnormal medical history or symptom that indicated I needed to be in hospital.

"Eleven and a half hours after she first arrived I gave birth to a healthy 6 lb 8 oz baby boy without any pain relief. I had no injections, no cuts, no stitches and I had a quiet, restful recovery for weeks afterwards."

Cathy Sykes

"I didn't plan to have my baby at home – I was registered with the community midwives to have her in hospital with their assistance.

"It started with pressure low down in the morning, and I thought she would be born that day. At lunchtime my membranes ruptured, in the kitchen fortunately, Alice and I had been to the Heathrow gym earlier. Initially it was a trickle and then it speeded up. I spent half an hour on the loo, letting it happen. I rang the community midwife's hotline and she came, tested it with a stick which turned black, to make sure it was amniotic fluid, and left. I rang my husband and my in-laws who came and took Alice away for the afternoon. I had a huge lunch because I was absolutely starving.

"The midwife came back a couple of times to check me – I pottered about, moaning about the Test Match and washing up and doing things to take my mind off it. Contractions got stronger and closer together and at 5 pm Donna said it was time to go in if we were going. By now the traffic would have built up and I couldn't face the thought of sitting in the car. The labour was progressing in a text-book fashion and it was obviously not going to take two days – unlike last time when it took twenty-four hours to get to 1 cm dilation. I was only comfortable sitting the wrong way round on a chair, leaning over the chair and it seemed ludicrous to make such an effort to get to hospital only to change rooms. Also I was terrified of being stuck on a monitor, which I had to have on all the time when I was having Alice.

"My midwife was quite happy to deliver the baby at home, I thought you would have to have masks and plastic everywhere, but my couple of old towels were enough, the midwives brought everything that was needed. She called her co-midwife who was just about to tuck into her tea not expecting to go out, and she kindly came bringing a huge cylinder of Entonox which my neighbour had to help her carry in.

"I got stuck into the Entonox, while the midwife read the *Property News*. Soon I wanted to push, and after a final check, I was able to do that. This time I was on all-fours instead of sitting up, and it was not long before Lucy was born. I infinitely preferred it that way, it was so much better.

"The nicest bit was yet to come, we were helped into a bath and then we were tucked up in bed. It could have been the seventeenth century – anytime, anywhere. The whole experience outshone the pain."

Wendy Primmer

"Babies are born in hospital. That's the normal way to do things, and it's not something to be questioned. Or so I thought . . .

"The first time my wife mentioned that she wanted a home birth I was more than a little sceptical. Being a scientist, it was clear to me that hospitals were best. Leave it to the professionals. Don't take any chances. Play it safe. I could see that persuading her out of the idea was going to be difficult, but I'd get her to see sense in the end. I'd start off by being really supportive and then slowly let her see the error of her ways until she could decide for herself that home birth was not for us. I was happy to be arrogant; naïve of the fact that I would be eating my own words soon enough.

"Whenever anyone found out that we were having a baby, they wanted to tell us their birth stories. How wonderful the event had been. What complications had arisen; most of them minor, others not quite so minor. It seemed that to one extent or another, each labour ended with the hospital staff doing an amazing job and saving the day. Hospital – safe. Home – unsafe.

"Over the summer, we attended the local NCT Home Birth Support Group. Each meeting brought together couples planning or thinking about home births for the purpose of sharing ideas and offering advice where needed. Every month one or two couples would return to the group with their newborn babies to talk about their recent birth stories. The contrast with the hospital births that I had heard was very noticeable. Both types of story talked about how hard it was; how much effort was involved; but the home birth stories were so much less dramatic. Midwives, family, and spouses were highly supportive, but nobody saved the day – there was no call for anything to be saved.

"And so I began questioning my original preconceived ideas. Why did the hospital stories all sound like a side plot from an episode of *Holby City*? Eventually, I started to notice a key point in each of the hospital birth stories. The story almost always seemed to change direction whenever some form of medical intervention was involved. Nobody ever seemed to question whether the intervention had been necessary or whether that was the cause of the resulting complications.

"I now believe that the first intervention occurs when you walk through the hospital doors. The relaxed atmosphere of home is lost and the alien environment of a maternity ward is entered causing nervousness and tension. At least, that's how I felt just going with my wife for a regular scan. Goodness knows how much more intense it is when you are in labour!

"My wife's first child was born when she was 26, in hospital after a series of interventions, finishing with a 22-stitch episiotomy. Her second child was born when she was 42, under water, at home after a 20 hour labour with no traditional pain relief, no drama and an intact perineum.

"I am clear now that nature knows far more about birth than medical science. If we stop interfering and let things go their own way at their pace the risks and complications are reduced significantly. As with everything in life, hospitals are ideal for emergency situations – it's just that most births aren't emergencies and don't need treating as such.

"I now believe that home water births are by far the best way to bring a child into the world. In my opinion, the home is the most relaxing place for a mother to give birth, and water offers the most effective form of pain relief whilst still retaining full control. I recommend it to anyone who wants as normal and simple a birth as possible."

Iain Anderson

6   obtaining a home birth

Despite misconceptions and misinformation, deliberate or otherwise, everyone has a legal right to have their baby at home. This applies whether it is your first, fourth, fifth or subsequent baby. It also applies if you are below average height, have complications in previous births, including forceps or Caesarean section, or if you have been told that you are at high risk of complications in this pregnancy. Obviously, a situation may arise where you might feel it is best to choose a hospital birth, but there is *no* category or situation that you can be in that makes it illegal for you to insist on your right to have your baby at home. However, it seems that health trusts are not obliged to provide a midwife to attend a woman wishing to give birth at home, although this may change. *You do not need to have a doctor's consent, nor do you need a doctor present at the birth.* The National Service Framework states that all women should have the option to contact a midwife as the first point of contact.

These are the options open to a woman wanting professional assistance with a home birth.

- **Doctor-only delivery.** A doctor is not bound to have a midwife present, although it is unusual for a doctor to want to deliver a baby at home single-handed.
- **Midwife-only delivery.** A midwife can deliver babies without calling anyone else, although some health authorities insist on a second midwife being present at delivery. A midwife may call on any doctor on the obstetric list to attend the delivery in an emergency or for suturing afterwards.
- **Doctor and midwife delivery.** The doctor consents to be responsible for medical care during the birth. In practice, however, although the doctor may be present, the midwife usually helps deliver the baby.

- **Independent midwife delivery.** You pay a private midwife to provide all your antenatal and postnatal care and to help you deliver the baby. She may work together with another independent midwife who will cover for her and provide services in an emergency.

GETTING A BOOKING

The way to get a home birth booking through any of the above routes is as follows.

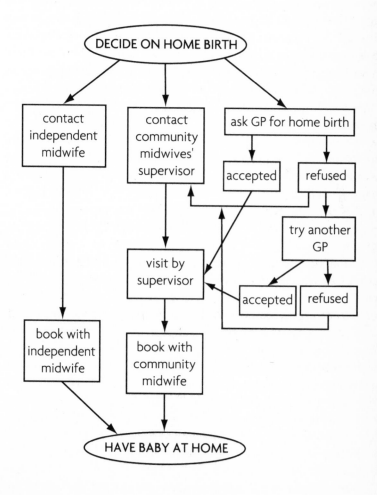

Options for booking a home birth

Doctor

It cannot be too strongly emphasised that you do not need to see your GP at all if you want to have your baby at home. You do not even have to let your doctor know that you are pregnant. Make the local Supervisor of Midwives (see below) the first person you contact once you know you want to have your baby at home.

It is probably only worth asking your doctor to be responsible for providing medical care for the birth of your baby in your home if you think that he or she is sympathetic to home birth or you particularly want him or her there. In either case go to your GP, say that you are pregnant and would like to have the baby at home. Be prepared for an unfavourable reaction. If it becomes clear that your doctor will not agree to attend, although he may offer to provide your antenatal and postnatal care, leave it there. Do not sign up for maternity care from your doctor unless you particularly want to have your antenatal care from both the doctor and the community midwives.

You can then, if you want, try another doctor that you know to be in favour of home birth. He or she can provide you with maternity care alone while you remain on your original doctor's list for anything not connected with the pregnancy.

Midwives

If your doctor refuses to provide you with medical care for home birth, or you do not want to ask your, or any other, doctor, or you would prefer all your maternity care from the midwives, apply to your local supervisor of midwifery services; you should be able to find her telephone number and address under Primary Health Care Trust under your local health authority listing in the phone book. Write to her stating when your baby is due, saying that you would like her to provide a midwife for antenatal care and delivery in your own home. Say that you accept full responsibility for your decision to give birth at home and that you know that they will accept the responsibility of providing you with a competent midwife fully backed up by such facilities as are necessary to make the birth as safe as possible.

There should be no argument about this, as the Government is committed to giving women the opportunity to have their babies at home. If you encounter problems contact the Association for Improvements in the Maternity Services (AIMS), **www.aims.org.uk**. They will be able to help you sort it out. It is also worth sending copies of your letter to the Chief Executive of your local trust, your Member of Parliament, your Local Supervisory Officer (see page 76). This will help to inform them of the demand for home births in your area. It is important to write rather than ring and to keep copies of all your letters and those you receive. You cannot rely on assurances made over the telephone.

Midwife and doctor delivery

You might have your antenatal care provided jointly by your doctor and the midwives. Your midwife will usually be with you for most of your labour and will just call the doctor for delivery. This will be arranged by your doctor.

Independent midwives and doula

The use of independent midwives and professional lay birth supporters, known as doulas, is growing. This may be because National Health Service support for home birth, although technically available, is currently uncertain. Women who want to be sure of having someone that they know with them at the birth, who believes in and has experience of home birth and who knows how to help a labouring women, may want to employ a professional birth attendant.

A doula cannot deliver a baby except in an emergency. An independent midwife is able to manage your antenatal care, help you have the baby and look after both of you postnatally. She may work on her own or with one or two other midwives. She is likely to see you in your home for antenatal visits, and she and/or one of her colleagues will be with you at the birth. Postnatal care may last up to six weeks. Independent midwives work as truly independent practitioners and have more freedom to exercise their professional judgement and are often able to take on 'high-risk' women. Although more midwives are choosing to work in this way, the numbers are relatively small and early booking is strongly recommended. Payment is by arrangement and there may be some flexibility about it.

Doulas (a Greek word meaning woman servant) may or may not be trained or registered. They may have been doing the job, unpaid, for many years. They provide emotional, physical, informational and practical support for the expectant, labouring or postpartum mother. A doula should be well-informed about current policies, best practice and local conditions. Some doulas provide day-to-day care for mothers and babies after the birth.

In employing an independent midwife or doula, you need to be certain that you are comfortable with each other. Ask around about her (NCT, Home Birth Support Group) and if possible take the opportunity to meet several.

You may want to discuss some of the following topics. Getting a sense of the way the person will be able to help you through birth, and feeling free to discuss your hopes and fears are the most vital aspects of meeting. In this, as in labour, it is important to trust your instinct.

- What service she provides – before, during and after birth. What are her fees and how does she want them paid?
- How long she has been doing it, how much experience she has of home birth, information about previous transfers. What does she enjoy about the job?
- Does she have any additional skills, e.g. reflexology, massage, acupuncture, herbs?
- Availability and contactability. Is the job shared with anyone else?
- What ifs? Talking through possible scenarios – both parties need to know the other person's position in various hypothetical situations. It is important that they will support your decisions, but they will want to be sure that you are aware of the possible risks and benefits of a particular choice. They will want to be sure that you realise that giving birth is hard work and that a given outcome cannot be guaranteed.
- Contact details of other mothers that have employed her.
- What happens next if you want to book her?

With luck you will take her on with a sense of excitement and anticipation, in the knowledge that she is willing and able to help you give birth in a way that you can look back on with pride.

ANTENATAL CARE

If you are booked with midwives for your delivery, you may get all your antenatal checks in your own home. Your booking visit should always be at home. In some cases you may then see the midwives in a local clinic or surgery. Be careful if you are asked to attend hospital, as this can be a way of getting you to change your mind. Make sure before you go that it is only on the understanding that you are booked for a home birth. You can refuse if you do not want to go. You do not need to see a consultant before being accepted for a home birth booking.

PROBLEMS

Of course all these things are all very well in theory, but the practice may be very different. Some women find that they have little or no trouble in booking a birth at home: others meet considerable opposition. It is as well to be prepared for this, because undoubtedly women sometimes do relinquish their chance of a home birth as a result of the pressure that is applied to them.

The reasons for these objections, the forms they take and the ways to circumvent them are as follows.

Doctors

Remember that you do not have to consult a doctor at all about having your baby at home. In fact not consulting one might be a wise precaution; GPs' reactions can be surprisingly fierce, even when such doctors are normally mild-mannered and considerate.

However, it is worth analysing the reasons for such reactions. In most cases it will not be a result of sheer bloody-mindedness, although it can seem like it. It can be due to apprehension and a genuine belief that you are proposing something that will endanger you and the baby and of course the doctor's reputation, notwithstanding the current evidence.

Part or all of this apprehension will stem from the doctor's previous experience of childbirth during his or her training, and may even go back further than that – to the type of person that he or she was before being selected for a place at medical school. In choosing science subjects a potential medical student is expressing a preference for subjects in which they study precise information and definite knowledge, rather than topics which are a matter of debate or interpretation. In a study in Toronto, medical students were compared with their contemporaries studying arts subjects. They scored more highly in intellect, achievement and endurance but substantially lower than the others in their ability to tolerate change, uncertainty and lack of structure. Clearly childbirth, with its unpredictable start, uncertain duration and emotional, uncontrolled nature, is unlikely to appeal to the average doctor.

Moreover, even those students starting medical school with a sensitive appreciation of people's needs find it difficult to maintain their sympathy in the rigidly conformist hospital atmosphere. They learn that it is more important not to make a mistake than to deal with people's emotional needs. They may be judged solely on results, and in childbirth the desired result is a healthy child, no matter what the cost in physical and psychological terms. In hospital the instruments are available for controlling the naturally untidy process of birth. Labour can be started at a convenient time, Syntocinon can limit its length and, should it fail to produce the desired result in the specified amount of time, ventouse, forceps or Caesarean section can bring the matter to a close. Although the doctor considers he is responsible for the outcome, there are others around with whom he can share the burden.

Interestingly, a study of the perceptions of pregnancy by obstetricians and midwives and pregnant women showed a difference in the degree of risk that each group thought it involved. Obstetricians, particularly males who had been practising longest, viewed pregnancy as being more risky than midwives, the longest-serving of whom regarded it as a normal event. Pregnant women saw it as being less risky than the obstetricians, although more risky than the midwives.[26]

Consider then the doctor's feelings if a woman comes to him rejecting this whole package and suggesting that she and her family are the ones responsible for the baby (whom he sees as his patient) and threatening him by asking him to deliver the baby without any of the support around him that he knows to be indispensable for safe delivery.

In any case his experience of any birth may be severely limited. He can qualify as a doctor having spent as little as seven days on the labour ward. He is most unlikely to have been with a pregnant woman from the time she is admitted to hospital until her baby is born. His experience of normal birth is likely to be limited to a brief dash into the room minutes before the birth; he is far more likely to have experience of the complicated delivery where midwives have been replaced by doctors. If he spent any time on the labour ward after qualifying he will have spent most of it making decisions about lack of progress, and acting on them, and performing ventouse, forceps and Caesarean section deliveries. He is most unlikely to have attended any home births except in alarming or unhappy circumstances such as a late miscarriage or secondary postpartum haemorrhage when the baby is a few days old, and again his impression will be of disaster attending home birth.

No wonder, then, that a request for a doctor to attend a home birth can alarm and frighten, to the extent that reason can fly out of the window. Such ingrained beliefs are unlikely to be altered by statistical evidence. The conclusion, then, is that you are better off without a doctor who agrees reluctantly and who is actually hoping for something to go wrong so that you have to go into hospital.

Women report frightening reactions from their doctors. They have been known to shout, to use emotional blackmail, to use threats that would be actionable if related to any other health area, and generally to make women feel very wretched and miserable at a time when they are feeling vulnerable anyway. They can also be deliberately misleading and say that women are not allowed to have their babies at home, e.g. if it is their first baby. It is true that there appears to be a greater acceptance of home birth as GP involvement decreases. It is also clear that GPs have a financial interest in providing maternity services – many women prefer to have all their care from midwives as it provides an opportunity to get to know them.

> "My doctor, with whom I normally get on well, took 40 minutes of surgery time to tell me that I would kill myself; she didn't care about me, but what about the baby? She gave me graphic descriptions of a ruptured uterus. She also used to ring me up at home to persuade me to change my mind and kept offering me more and more concessions if I would consent to go in – even ultimately a woman consultant visiting me at home."

Sometimes doctors feel ambivalent about helping you, or they may offer ante and postnatal care but refuse to cover you for the birth. Others may refer you to another doctor. Some feel so strongly about the subject that they strike you off their register. (You cannot be struck off if you have already signed on for maternity care unless it is with your consent or the doctor applies to the family practitioner committee. If he or she strikes you off without either your or their consent, he is in breach of contract and should be reported to the Primary Care Trust straight away.)

However, you cannot force your doctor to cover you for the birth, and you probably would not want to anyhow. If you decide to choose a midwife delivery then it is probably best to get all your antenatal care from the community midwives; they can refer you to a consultant in the event of a problem.

Midwives

Opting for delivery by your community midwives is not necessarily straightforward. Local health trusts vary in their enthusiasm for providing a home birth service, so that near neighbours may get a completely different service. The midwives, from the most senior, the director of midwifery services, downwards may feel obliged to deter you, either as a result of their own beliefs or because they are so instructed by their health authority policy. It seems likely that there would be many more home births if women were given a real choice in the matter, but all too frequently they find it difficult to ask for one or find that, if they do, they are further put off by the attitude of the midwife they first speak to.

It may be that the policy in your area is one of discouraging home birth and that a midwife knows that booking you for home birth will be frowned upon either by her seniors or by her colleagues. Even within an area which is well disposed to home birth, different community midwives feel differently about the subject. Some will really relish it and be positive about it. These midwives are keen to be present at the birth and will go out of their way to be there on the day. They are undoubtedly midwives who have experience of home birth and who have learnt through observation that birth goes better at home.

Others, either hospital midwives or those whose experience of community work is limited, or who work for an authority that positively discourages home birth, are likely to feel negative about it. Again, training is responsible.

Recently qualified UK midwives should have a degree in midwifery. Previously, some midwives went directly into midwifery training but the majority began their training after three years training to be nurses. As one experienced community midwife, who is a firm believer in home birth, explained:

"So that means that midwives are primarily nurses. They have been trained in care which involves assisting in every bodily function. They are trained to observe functions minutely – they are not just interested in bowels but assist them to move. They are not just interested in sputum but have to note the amount, colour and consistency. If things are not appropriate then the nurse is taught to take action to change them.

"When it comes to midwifery they are trained in the same way. They note fluid intake, they control it by denying women drinks in labour and then hydrating her with a drip; they then observe her urinary output, test it and measure it. They learn how to manage labour.

"They learn to position her in bed, take routine observations without question. They offer mandatory pain relief, offer antiemetics and intravenous fluids instead of food. They treat the woman as sick and prepare her for operative delivery.

"They manage pregnancy by not informing women what is going on, by not encouraging them to carry their notes. The midwife is trained to take over all functions and responsibility. When she does then the woman thinks 'Let her get on with it' and then the midwife shares the woman's belief in her control.

"As a result of this training midwives find it very hard to let go and allow the woman to take control. Home birth is seen as admitting defeat because she, the midwife, has to relinquish control. In fact it is noticeable that women booking for home birth are quite different in their attitude. They are usually acutely aware of their own bodies and very aware that going into hospital means giving up their fundamental rights.

"If midwives learnt from women, rather than through their training and obstetricians, they would learn to trust them and their judgement. If midwives feel comfortable about home delivery the midwives should learn to trust that feeling. It usually means that the midwives would have to give a lot of themselves in terms of time, warmth, love and trust. Being with woman (the literal meaning of midwife) shouldn't mean being present with her in body and taking over all her functions; it should mean with the woman in the midwife's mind, understanding what she is going through and encouraging her in her natural process. The woman must know that she can trust the midwife, that she really does know what is happening to her, so that she believes in her strength to see her through."

Another community midwife pointed out that midwives can be anxious about home birth because it is not adequately covered in their training. A midwife may qualify having been present at only one or two home births, if she is lucky. A qualified midwife can therefore find herself in the position of delivering a baby at home, never having done it before. Without an inherent belief in women's ability to give birth unaided – a belief she will not gain in hospital – she, as well as the doctor, can be terrified by the prospect.

Not only might a midwife feel inadequately trained to cope with birth at home, but she, even more than a doctor, is also subject to hierarchical pressure. In terms of power and authority the midwife is almost at the bottom of the ladder (while the mother has not even got her feet on it) and she is answerable to her supervisor, the director of midwifery services, and to any doctor, consultants in particular. She also has to maintain a working relationship with her colleagues, whom she will still be seeing long after your baby is born. If the majority of these people see home birth as professional suicide, it is going to take a lot of courage to book you for home birth, even if she is basically sympathetic.

This is why you have to be adamant about your decision. Unless you only meet with a favourable response, you need to be completely firm about your decision. Although it is a pity not to have the opportunity to discuss the pros and cons freely with your midwife, you can only be sure of getting what you want by presenting an assured front.

Even if you decide to have a midwife-only delivery and you write and request this, you may find that you are visited by a senior midwife. She has a duty to make sure that you understand the implications of your decision. She may also want to discourage you, so that it is as well to be prepared to have your views challenged.

It can be unnerving to have someone arrive on your doorstep, either with or without an appointment, so it may help to remember that, because she is coming into your home, you have the advantage. If you are fortunate you will have an amicable discussion about having the baby at home and she will agree to book you, although perhaps with some show of reluctance. At worst you will be subject to intense pressure to change your mind. The sort of means sometimes employed by doctors and midwives include the following examples:

- What will happen if something goes wrong and your baby dies. How will you feel then?
- What will happen if you die?
- If you'd ever seen a postpartum haemorrhage you would never risk such a thing.
- What if you needed the ambulance and they were dealing with someone who was dying?
- Wouldn't you feel guilty if you took the ambulance from the hospital where those people are needed?
- You know you can't have an epidural at home.
- We have had a stillbirth at home in our practice (the mother was booked for a hospital delivery).

The above examples are quite unpleasant but non-specific. In some ways more worrying are the threats which are applied to you directly. In this category can come some very misleading assessments of your childbearing ability based on theoretical or inaccurate information. For example:

- Your obstetric history is poor.
- You are not allowed to have your first baby at home.
- Your blood pressure is too high (without evidence).

Another technique that is used is the conditional refusal, e.g. 'Well, we would consider it if it was your second baby/you hadn't had forceps last time/you were taller, younger, etc.' These exasperating provisos are just excuses, though. Almost no one is going to fit into the stereotype of an 'ideal' home-birth candidate implied by these suggestions. Even if you were a supported mother expecting her second or third child, above 5 feet 1 inch in height, between the ages of 23 and 30, with a blameless obstetric history, immaculate home conditions, with your mother to hand, then there would still probably be something that would render you 'unsuitable this time, perhaps next time dear'.

Some women find it easy to deal with this pressure. They simply do not see a problem. They ask for what they want, are not interested in the objections and get what they ask for. Many of us, however, have been brought up to accept authority; especially that of the medical profession, and as women have learnt to be compliant. It can therefore be difficult to hold out for what you want, especially if you are having to defend your choice when you may be feeling more than ordinarily emotional and vulnerable. However committed you may be to home birth, you are bound to have some doubts. No one can know exactly how labour will progress, and most women meet at least with some lack of approval over their decision from family or friends. This can leave you open to suggestion when objections are put powerfully by a doctor or midwife. Insisting on your rights can be difficult, particularly when those trying to deny you them are more experienced in this type of negotiation than you.

If you find it hard then you may want to employ assertion techniques to get what you want. Put into practice, these can be very effective. It is very helpful to practise them before you need to use them, perhaps by role-playing the imagined scene in advance with a friend.

If you can, have your partner or a friend with you at the interview. Have the points you wish to make written down on a list in advance. Avoid any such meeting away from your own territory if possible. If the doctor or midwife is really keen to talk you out of home birth, they will agree to visit you at home, where you will be more at ease than they are. It is important not to agree to visit those who may put further pressure on you, such as a consultant, or to book for a hospital birth 'just in case'.

Assume from the start that your views are going to be respected. Appear confident and assured (even if you don't feel it). Ensure that you are not at a physical disadvantage, for example flat on your back being examined or partially dressed, or in a chair that is lower than your opponents. If the doctor or midwife tries to start a discussion while you are at such a disadvantage, just say that you would prefer to discuss it when you are dressed, or whatever.

Speak directly and clearly, dealing with the easiest part of your request first. Take a deep breath, and maintain eye contact. Appear relaxed and confident. Be open and honest about what you want; remember, you are only asking for a service that the Government says you should have. Make sure that you listen to the replies and that you acknowledge them, without being side-tracked, e.g. 'Thank you for your concern, I appreciate that you think that home birth is dangerous, but I would still prefer to have my baby at home.'

Remember that the other party has rights too, and that they are trying to do what they see as the best for you. If they genuinely think that you are not safe giving birth except in hospital, then they are fearful for you as well as themselves. Always speak pleasantly and calmly, without becoming angry, upset or aggressive. Make it clear that you are not attacking them, only disagreeing with what is proposed.

If reasoned discussion is failing to achieve your aim, then you can fall back on the 'scratched record' technique. This is an astonishingly effective way of getting what you want, but it is important to try it out beforehand, both so that you become familiar with it and also so that you can appreciate how powerful it is. It involves stating what you want simply and repeatedly, even if your request is not acknowledged.

"I want to have my baby at home."
"I know you think that now but I don't think you really realise what it involves. After all no birth can be said to be safe until it is over and you know how far you live from the hospital. What would happen if you suddenly started to bleed badly after the birth or the baby had problems? After all, at your age problems are much more likely you know."
"Yes, thank you for your concern, I appreciate that you do not think it is a good idea, but I still want to have my baby at home."
'Don't you think that you are being rather selfish, just wanting a home birth for your own satisfaction. I mean you might be all right and it might be lovely for you, but you are putting your baby's life at risk. Have you thought of that? I mean, someone has got to look after the baby's interests, it can't speak for itself.

It could be brain-damaged if things go wrong here. Why don't you consider a domino delivery; it wouldn't normally be available to you but I think we could make a special concession in your case."

"Thank you for your offer, but I still want to have my baby at home."

"You know, it's very inconvenient, you're asking for a lot of time and commitment from my midwives and they are sorely over-stretched as it is. I see you had forceps and epidural last time; how do you know you won't need them again? I mean, you can't have an epidural at home you know. And Mr Bloggs the consult-ant is very opposed to home births. I doubt that you could count on his assistance when you need him in an emergency."

"I'm sorry if you find it inconvenient, but I still want to have my baby at home."

"Well as you know, we are legally obliged to take on even the most unsuitable cases, unlike doctors who can select whom they take on for home birth. I think you are being most unwise, and this is against my professional judgement, but if you are not pre-pared to change your mind, and as long as you realise that you are fully responsible for your actions, I will send a midwife to book you for home birth. I trust that you will accept a hospital delivery if there should be the slightest indication of anything untoward. You know that you can change your mind at anytime."

"Yes, thank you very much. I appreciate the trouble you've taken."

WOMEN'S STORIES

You really do need to be forewarned and forearmed, because the way in which a request for a home birth is handled can be enough to deter you. This will probably be deliberate, and includes unjusti-fiable scaremongering, 'forgetting' your request, ignoring it and booking you for a hospital delivery instead, making you an appoint-ment either to see the consultant or for a scan so that the hospital staff can talk you out of it, outright blackmail and harassment. These forms of persuasion should end once you have got your home birth booking, but unfortunately there is evidence that in some cases pressure is maintained. Women are sometimes told that they are suffering from complications of pregnancy that necessitate hospital delivery when this is not the case. It would be nice to believe that it cannot be true, but some doctors and midwives do believe that the end justifies the means. The trouble is that if they have already lost your respect and trust, you can no longer be sure that they are telling you the truth. Some stories will illustrate these points.

"He [the GP] commented that home births just do not happen these days and they are terrifyingly dangerous events. My experience is different but obviously one gets demoralised when such comments are made and I am beginning to get cold feet before I have even started."

Heather Heales (Heather has now had two babies at home)

"I was 12 weeks pregnant when it was discovered, and after my first antenatal appointment I noticed I had been put down for a hospital birth . . . At my next appointment I expressed a desire for a home birth and tried to explain to my GP my reasons. Although he admitted he was not happy with my request he said if it was what I wanted it could be arranged. Needless to say I was extremely relieved and started to enjoy the thought of the birth.

"At 20 weeks pregnant I had to see the obstetrician, and she knew nothing about my request. After enquiring, she informed me that my GP had done nothing about my request because he did not want me to have a home birth and he hoped I would change my mind, especially if nothing was mentioned about it. To say the least I was both amazed and upset, and arranged to see my GP.

"Again he expressed the fact that he was unhappy about it, but if it was what I really wanted he would arrange it. He also said I would not have to find another GP practice for the birth. That was when I was 20 weeks pregnant.

"Last week I went for my 28-week antenatal appointment and it was another GP (still from the same practice). The subject of home birth came up and the GP said nothing had been said to him about it, and for a home birth all the GPs of the practice should be told and agree to it. On enquiring, he was told by the midwife that nothing had been done because my usual GP was hoping I would change my mind as the birth comes closer.

"At the moment I don't know where to go from here and I feel disgust at the way my request was handled – my pregnancy has been turned into a distasteful experience and the thought of a hospital birth has me resenting the medical profession and filled with an uncomfortable fear. Also certain things have been said to me by both my GP and midwife that have lowered my respect and trust in them, and each antenatal appointment is becoming more of an ordeal than a comfort."

Joan Davis (see birth report on page 71)

"My situation at present is that my doctor is unwilling to provide cover for a home birth and the community midwife whom I met tried in an almost threatening manner to dissuade me, stating 'We do not do home births here.'"

"I had my first antenatal check-up this morning at the local hospital and voiced my desire for a home birth to the consultant. I couldn't believe his response – he acted as if I had absolutely no say over the birth, that I was acting 'irresponsibly' and that there is no way he is going to allow a home birth. I left the hospital in tears, but even more determined to get my way."

Karen Condon (see birth report on page 40)

"I have reached the point where I am just about to give up trying to fight the system in this area as I am meeting so many brick walls and none of the medical profession seems to have any confidence in attending births. I am afraid that I am running out of strength to fight them all and being 30 weeks pregnant now I have to confess to feeling vulnerable and I hate having to admit that."

"I suffered a miscarriage. The next year I fell pregnant again – I contacted my doctor and had the pregnancy confirmed. I was very worried as I was having a discharge and thought once again I might miscarry, so you can imagine how upset I was when my doctor said he thought the baby had died but as yet I hadn't miscarried. He said he would arrange a scan (for which I had to wait eight weeks) and if by chance I was still pregnant, he would only see me again if I would agree to have the baby in hospital. I never saw him again until after the baby was born (at home)."

E. M. Court

"I saw my regular GP, Dr X. He exploded when I said I would like to have a home birth.

"I then went to see the highly recommended consultant Mr Y. The clinic he ran was appalling, overcrowded and had inhuman treatment as a result. When I finally got to see him, his first word or words were 'Couch' – he meant for me to get on the couch. However I thought he was referring to an animal, not me, so I sat down on the chair and asked if I could speak to him first. I remained pleasant and controlled. I mentioned home birth and he and three nurses and one other doctor present in the room had a field day intimidating me. I was told no doctor would give me cover (even though I knew I didn't need it), no doctor would come out after 5 pm, my child would probably be deformed if born at home, etc., etc., that there was something wrong with my pelvis which would make it impossible for a home delivery. Needless to say I left in tears.

"That was when the information from the home birth support group arrived. I wrote the letter they suggested and received a reply saying arrangements were being made.

"I then had a phone call from a Nurse Z asking me why I wanted the child at home, why don't I go to the hospital to discuss it, what about the pelvis, who was the GP who was going to cover me?

"That was it, I had had enough. I contacted AIMS, NMC, Beverley Beech, and MIDIRS. They put me straight and calmed me down. They were very helpful and told me to contact them with any further problems. After that I insisted that they came round to me. There have been no further problems – so far – although my trust and faith in the profession will never be fully restored. . . . I subsequently saw a doctor privately who said there was nothing wrong with my pelvis."

Deborah Wilson (see birth report on page 125)

"My GP was prepared to deliver my baby at home. The midwife I saw at an antenatal clinic advised against it. She duly informed the obstetrician of my intentions and I was treated appallingly by him.

"I was made to feel like I was a witness in a crown court. He got quite angry and questioned me again and again about the exact words of my GP. He said he was very angry with my GP and that he would be writing to him. Then in a fancy obstetrician way he as much as told me that if I decide to go ahead with this crazy idea then he would have nothing more to do with me. I came out of his consulting room in tears and heartbroken. Completely open-minded, I was prepared to listen to his medical advice, I argued my case calmly and coolly in an educated manner. Frankly I was shocked by his manner. The midwife told me that he wasn't used to having his authority questioned or dealing with educated women, and that he had 'gone over the top' with me."

Karen Parkinson

"I wanted to have my third baby at home and, after being refused by one practice, was accepted a doctor at another. That was fine until 38 weeks when that same doctor called at my home at 8 am to tell me he had nearly lost a mother and child in a GP unit and that I should think hard before going ahead with 'this idea'.

"My husband rang this doctor and told him that we intended to go ahead with a home birth. Unfortunately however a late scan showed a slightly low-lying placenta, so of course we had to give in to the pressure, despite the fact that at 39½ weeks my midwife reported that the placenta had slipped back out of the way."

"These were the reasons given by my health visitor:
- I simply would not be allowed a home birth.
- No midwife would agree to call.
- I should not antagonise the doctors – I would no doubt risk being labelled a troublemaker and be blacklisted nationally.
- I would probably die, or at best the baby would.
- As I don't know my new address, I may have to change midwives, again if I find a midwife to 'agree' in the first place (I don't understand this one either). In response I told her that, as it was my right and not at the whim of the area health authority whether I had a home birth, I failed to see

her point.

- She also told me that, should I persist and then require a doctor to attend my children, they may be subject to bullying by the doctor. I told her any such behaviour would naturally be brought to the attention of the Family Practitioners' Committee in writing."

"I realise that my age (35) and this being my first baby leads the medical profession to advise a hospital delivery, but no account seems to be taken of my psychological state. Even antenatal visits to the hospital leave me tense, anxious and drained, not due to the staff there but to my own feelings about it.

"I had no wish to antagonise anyone over this and realise the importance of trying to gain their understanding, but feel I am getting nowhere. . . .

"My own doctor is someone I feel confident of and feel he is a caring and competent man. Unfortunately he has not delivered a baby for eight years and is unwilling to cover the midwives at a home delivery. He has tried to find a GP to take me on but seems to have had no success and we seem to have reached something of an impasse. I see the consultant at the hospital alternately with attending the midwives clinic at the local surgery.

"I am beginning to feel very isolated over this matter and am almost afraid to approach anyone for fear of yet another browbeating over how stupid I am being. My husband respects my wishes, but is being constantly accosted by people who 'wouldn't let my wife do it' and telling him tales of death, gloom and gore. . . ."

Jackie Reay (see birth report on page 171)

"He also said it could take up to one and a half hours for the paramedics to get here if there was an emergency, which seems ridiculous. My local maternity hospital is only about seven minutes drive away."

"I am the 37-year-old mother of a three-year-old boy who was born by Caesarean section. This occurred because I was two weeks overdue and under great pressure to be induced, which

I was very much opposed to. The section took place after 18 hours of labour by which time I was deemed to have 'failed to progress'. My waters had leaked at home with slight meconium staining, but the baby's heartbeat was fine. I was 3 cm dilated at home and very happy and self-assured and excited, but when the midwife insisted after three hours that we go to hospital I stopped dilating. After eight hours I was pressured into having Syntocinon 'for the sake of the baby'. I only dilated a further 3 cm after 10 more hours and then it was strongly urged that I had a Caesarean with an epidural. I had instinctively been against having an epidural, but in this, as in all that had preceded the labour so far, I swallowed my feelings and was compliant. For 20 minutes they tried to find the right place for the needle, to no avail. All the while I was having powerful Syntocinon contractions and the only pain relief I would accept was the TENS and Entonox. It ended with a general anaesthetic. The following day it transpired that I had a dural tap headache and was in blinding pain for six days and required total bedrest. My son was in special care for five days for observation of a stomach infection which was the result of his fetal distress. My husband and I had been left for hours and hours alone and unsupported. When people did come in it was to intervene with medical means and take the experience away from us. No one suggested ways we could do it better – we felt more and more helpless and passive and unempowered with each intervention.

"It took me weeks, if not months, to stop feeling depressed and anxious and disconnected from my son. As soon as I began to feel better I put the whole event behind me and worked hard at being positive and looking forward.

"When I became pregnant again two years and two months later, I still thought very little about the previous labour until I was about two months pregnant. I then read an American book called *The Vaginal Birth After Caesarean Experience* by Lyn Baptisti Richards, which turned my life upside down and put me in touch with all the repressed feelings of distress and anger about the first birth. It was very painful but important to rant and rave and grieve for all the awful experience my son and I had gone through. I reached out to a particular midwife to help me understand and make sense of what had happened in the previous labour. She was very helpful and gave me the name and number of an NCT teacher who proved to be an invaluable support and ally. The NCT teacher offered to be present at the birth and supported us all along in many different ways leading up to the birth. During the course of our discussions we all began to embrace the idea of a home birth, and this grew and grew until it became a wish very dear to my heart.

"By this time it was four weeks before the baby was due. A young innovative GP agreed to attend me at home and the community midwives very reluctantly agreed to my home birth. It took a lot of energy setting the whole thing up and my spirits would soar and dip daily as people either blocked or encouraged me. I was very apprehensive about telling my GP and it wasn't until three and a half weeks before the due date that I did tell her. Her negative and punitive response was very powerful and sent me reeling and shaking for a good two days; being shouted at and told I was selfish, putting myself before baby, too old, carrying too big a baby, likely to have a disabled child, in the care of an inexperienced GP who was acting irresponsibly plus in the care of midwives who were 'only nurses', shook me to the core. She demanded to know what reasons I had for such a foolish wish, but it did not feel that she was really interested, only looking for more holes to poke in any argument I might have.

"She insisted upon speaking to the GP who was willing to attend me and, out of fairness to the latter GP, I agreed. My GP somewhat frightened the younger GP and from that point on I felt at pains to reassure her and thereby lost her as the full support I had initially experienced. Basically I was very disappointed and surprised at my GP's total lack of understanding and appreciation at how open and vulnerable a pregnant woman can be."

Sally

(Sally later had a little girl, Daniella, in hospital because she developed a high fever and consequently went into labour. She was able to push her out with the aid of forceps after a long labour with which she coped well.)

"With regard to the rest of my pregnancy, at the next visit to my GP they were very helpful about my request for a home birth. (The GP I had seen on my previous visit was one of the senior practitioners and I believe he had something to do with the change of attitude of my GP.) I was told that as long as I was past 37 weeks of my term I could have my child at home.

"The midwife came out to the house and said that everything was fine with regards to the position of the bed, the amount of room she had to work in, the tables that she would need. She kept mentioning the 'mess' there would be, and that she was concerned about not having the necessary equipment if the baby's heart stopped or if she stopped breathing after birth. Then she'd say that she supposed it was easy to resuscitate a baby. She mentioned everything that could go wrong and how concerned she was that it would take twenty or thirty minutes to get the baby to hospital. It struck me as really weird how in the antenatal classes she was minimising the risks and things that could go wrong, but with me at home, she was the opposite. I felt she was deliberately trying to 'worry me' into a hospital birth, instead of helping me to relax and enjoy my pregnancy. She arranged to bring everything she needed to the house the day before I would be 37 weeks.

"I went into labour at five in the morning the day before I was 37 weeks – the same day the midwife was to bring everything to my house. I rang the hospital at about 6.30 in the morning and they rang the midwife. She phoned me and said she had nothing for pain relief and no way of getting any. Also, since I was not yet 37 weeks, I had to go in.

"So I went to hospital and as I arrived there the shifts were changing and I had to wait for 10-15 minutes before being examined. By that time I was dilated to 7 cm and I was told the only thing I could have for pain relief was the 'gas and air'. I was not in any pain and after the contractions using the gas and air I was told to push. Jacqueline was born at 9.28 that morning with no cutting or stitching required and the experience was not painful in any way.

"Shortly afterwards the midwife who had looked after me during my pregnancy came to see me and told me she'd had gas and air in her car, so I could have had Jacqueline at home. I would have liked the choice earlier when she told me to go to hospital."

Joan Davis

THE LEGAL POSITION ON HOME BIRTH

At the time of writing the original and subsequent editions of this book it was believed by both parents and providers that there was a legal responsibility to provide a home birth service under the NHS. However, as carefully described by Nadine Pilley Edwards in her book, *Birthing Autonomy*, it was discovered as a result of an editorial article in *Practising Midwife* that because the term 'domiciliary' was omitted from the NHS Act of 1977, women did not in fact have a legal right to services for labour outside hospital. As a consequence some NHS trusts began to withdraw their domiciliary services so that the current position is that women are entitled to choose to have their babies at home, the Government[27] is encouraging women to have their babies at home, the NICE guidelines suggest that planning birth at home increases the chances of having a normal birth and that women should be given the choice over where they give birth, but in practice there is no guarantee that the local health authority will supply a midwife when a woman calls in when she is in labour.

Evidence collected from around the UK by AIMS shows that the practice of sending a letter to women booked for home birth stating that the trust/providers may not be able to provide cover for home birth is common. This letter (see example) is often sent at around 37 weeks of pregnancy – although it may be sent or given earlier.

Dear
    You have requested to have your baby, due [date], at home.
    As there is a high rise in births across the area for the foreseeable future you should be aware that it might not be possible for a midwife to come to you at home. This will be because midwives are unable to be released from the maternity unit and the workload there. In this rare event you will be asked to come into the hospital for the birth of your baby.
    Whilst we fully understand the disappointment this may cause we have to do this for safety reasons for yourself, your baby and for other women who require the attention of midwives in the maternity unit.
    We hope that should you be asked to do this you will co-operate and come into the unit. Not to do so will put yourself

and your baby at risk. We will aim to get you home again as soon as possible, probably within 6 hours of your baby's birth.

We apologise for any inconvenience this may cause.

Supervisor of Midwives

In March 2006, the Nursing and Midwifery Council (the midwives professional body) issued a circular[28] making it clear among other things that a midwife's professional duty of care is to the woman in her charge and that she should treat her with competence or else find someone who can. Should there be a dispute between her duty to her employers and her duty to a woman in her care, her care of the woman should take precedence. This is valuable information for both women and midwives.

On confidence and competence

It may be that a midwife does not have the experience required to care for a particular woman at home. In order to fulfil her duty of care she may:

- Take steps to update her own knowledge and skills to gain such experience so she can support the woman
- Seek help from her manager or supervisor of midwives to gain support to do this
- If time is limited, refer the care of this woman to colleagues who have the competence, then take steps to update herself to ensure she becomes competent for the future.

On risk

Risk is a complex issue; however there is no system currently available in the maternity services, which helps elicit absolute risk or accurately predicts adverse outcome.

It is a midwife's duty to make all options and choices clear and to respect the choices a woman makes if she is legally competent to make that choice.

On resources

Should a conflict arise between service provision and a woman's *choice for place of birth, a midwife has a duty of care to attend her. This is no different to a woman who has walked into a mater-nity unit to receive hospital care. Withdrawal of a home birth serv-ice is no less significant to women than withdrawal of services for a hospital birth.*

The situation is currently fluid – despite official backing for home birth from NHS Direct, NICE and the NMC, it seems as hard or harder to be sure of having a midwife come to your home to help you give birth. The anxiety that this causes can be considerable. For these reasons, as well as to improve the home birth service for the future, it seems as though it would be valuable to write (do not ring, it is important to have everything in writing) to your Supervisor of Midwives (address through your local hospital) as soon as you know that you are pregnant and want to have your baby at home. It will help her to plan, and evidence from AIMS suggests that the earlier you make your wishes known the greater the chance of your achieving them. You might like to write some-thing along the lines of:

Dear Supervisor,
    I am expecting a baby on [due date] and intend to give birth at home. I have studied the NICE guidelines on the safety of home birth and appreciate that 'planning birth at home increas-es the likelihood of a normal vaginal birth and satisfaction in women who are committed to giving birth in this setting com-pared to planning birth in hospital'.
    I would be grateful if you would arrange for me to receive antenatal and labour care from a midwife who is experienced in, and confident about, helping women to give birth at home.
    With thanks, yours, etc.

Should you then get the letter (see page 73) or if you have not been in contact with the supervisor prior to getting the letter, it is suggested that you write immediately to the Supervisor of Midwives along the following lines:

Dear [name],
    I have received a letter from [name] stating that I may not be provided with intrapartum midwifery care when I am in labour

at home due to midwifery shortages.

As you are aware it is Government policy to encourage home births and the NICE guidelines state that everyone should be able to choose where to give birth provided that they are fully informed about the potential risks and benefits of each birth setting. I am also aware that NMC guidelines (March 2006) state that 'should a conflict arise between service provision and a woman's choice of place of birth, a midwife has a duty of care to attend her'.

I am committed to giving birth at home, so please would you ensure that there is a competent midwife experienced in assisting at home birth available to attend me at home over the period my baby is due. I do not intend to have my baby in hospital unless complications prior to or during my labour make it necessary.

Yours, etc.

AIMS suggests: 'Send copies of your letter to the following people, together with a covering letter asking them to help you.

- Beverley Beech, Chair of AIMS (see Useful Addresses).
- The Chief Executive of your local trust (his or her name may be on the letter that you received).
- Your Member of Parliament.
- Your Local Supervisory Authority Officer.

'Every area has a Local Supervising Authority (LSA) Responsible Officer. She is a senior midwife who is responsible for midwifery practice in your area and we suggest contacting her; she can lean on the Trust. You can find out her address from the Director of Midwifery's secretary, or by telephoning the Nursing and Midwifery Council.

'It is also very worthwhile contacting the local press, and if you want to give them the number of the AIMS Chair, Beverley Beech, Tel 0870-765 1433, she will give them further information and quotes. Contacting the press will also alert other women in the area who are faced with the same problem.'

It is AIMS' experience that making your stance clear in writing in this way, will ensure that you are supplied with a midwife. However it is also true that women are still being told to come into hospital when in labour and that they cannot legally stay at home. This perhaps refers to the question of it being unlawful (see page 149). It is obviously quite untrue that it is illegal for a woman to stay at home while she is giving birth even if those responsible feel unable to send a midwife to her.

Should this happen to you say that you are unable to move and ask a midwife to attend as a matter of urgency and make it clear that you are not coming in. If they still refuse, ask for the name and status of the person you are speaking to (it should be you, the labouring woman, making the request) and ask if they will send an ambulance with paramedics to help you give birth at home.

This situation is very far from ideal and extremely hard on women in labour – it is far better, if at all possible, to have ensured already that that a viable home birth service is running at all times. It is this sort of anxiety that makes people choose the services of an independent midwife (see page 53).

SPECIAL NOTE: DISCLAIMERS

You may be asked to sign a disclaimer accepting full responsibility for giving birth at home and absolving the health authority of any culpability in the event of anything going wrong. Such declarations have no legal standing and would not mean that the authority could not be held responsible if anything went wrong as a result of negligence on their behalf. You are under no obligation to sign although, of course, you can if you wish, perhaps writing underneath that you understand it is not legally binding.

AIMS would like copies of any such notes.

7 the high-risk pregnancy

"Don't forget us high-risk mothers."

Getting a booking to have your baby at home can be hard enough for a woman of average height, expecting her second child after a perfectly straightforward first labour. If, as is likely, you fall outside this very specific category, then you can expect even greater objections based on your allegedly 'high-risk' status.

Many doctors will consider you to be at high risk of experiencing complications in pregnancy or labour if you are:

- Expecting your first baby.
- Expecting a fourth, fifth or subsequent baby.
- Are 30 or older if it's your first baby, or older than 35 if you already have a child.
- You have had an operation on your uterus, including Caesarean section.
- You had a ventouse or forceps delivery last time.
- You are under 5 feet 1 inch tall.
- You have previously had a postpartum haemorrhage.

In many cases these objections will be related to statistical risk rather than directly to you. Independent midwives have a strong belief in the benefits of home births and consider that very few conditions render a woman unsuitable to have her baby at home. They find that a healthy lifestyle and an informed, positive attitude is likely to result in a successful home birth, regardless of the mother's age or her previous history. Their attitude of encouragement and belief in a woman's ability to give birth unaided means that women under their care do just that, even though they may be deemed to be at very high risk of encountering problems.

In some instances it is quite clear that refusal by a doctor to accept you for home delivery because you fit into one of these categories is due merely to a reluctance to do any home deliveries; for example, the woman who was turned down because she was 'too short' at 5 feet 1¾ inches.

If you are fit, healthy and taking positive steps to ensure the health of yourself and your baby, these factors can become irrelevant. The most pertinent objections are those related to your particular obstetric history. You will have to decide whether previous problems arose because of circumstances which remain the same in this pregnancy, e.g. contracted pelvis (where the pelvis is deformed due to injury or illness); or whether they could have been due to the way your labour was handled or were specific to that individual baby. For example, the previous problems might have arisen because your labour was actively managed, because you felt tense or inhibited in hospital surroundings or with unhelpful staff, or because the baby became distressed. If you are uncertain as to whether circumstances will repeat themselves, you have to choose between having the baby in hospital or booking for a home delivery bearing in mind the possibility of transfer. If you opt for home but have to go in, you will at least know that the need for hospitalisation has been demonstrated and that you are less likely to be subject to 'just-in-case' obstetrics. On the other hand, you do have to be able to feel that you can trust your attendants, as it is in precisely this sort of situation that a midwife or doctor who has doubts about home birth will err on the side of conservatism and get you transferred. There is also the very relevant point that negative emotions and lack of enthusiasm will have a detrimental effect on your labour and justify their fears.

Some conditions will be unique to you so that only you will be able to weigh them up and come to a decision. However the following guidelines can be offered, together with some suggestions as to their validity.

HEIGHT

It is helpful to know that smaller women can and do give birth at home without problems — see page 90. Women generally have babies to fit them, added to which the pelvis also increases in diameter during labour.

One practitioner claims that 'supine and semi-recumbent

labour positions tend to close the pelvis, denying mother and fetus up to 30 per cent of pelvic outlet area.'[29]

AGE

This is irrelevant if you are healthy. Statistics showing that women do less well obstetrically as they get older include all those whose labour has been actively managed because of their age and who have consequently had instrumental deliveries. It also includes those who have had large numbers of children while in poor health with short intervals between births.

FIRST, OR FOURTH OR SUBSEQUENT BABY

This should not disqualify anyone from having their baby at home. Labour usually takes longer for a first baby and there is a higher incidence of transfer, although this may reflect the attitude of the attendants (see the example on page 177 where the midwife had said that none of her mothers achieved a first birth at home). Home birth is likely to be especially suitable for later babies in the family, when labour may well be very rapid (page 86). NICE guidelines suggest birth in a consultant-led unit for fifth and subsequent babies.

HOME CONDITIONS

Ideally a home should be clean, warm and have running water. It is helpful, but not essential, to have a phone. Some of the stipulations made by midwives such as that the bathroom must be on the same floor as the bedroom are unnecessary.

It is possible to give birth anywhere – babies that arrive without warning are born safely in some very unsuitable places, such as cars and car parks.

PREVIOUS OBSTETRIC DIFFICULTIES

This objection will depend very much on what happened before, but need not necessarily be discouraging, even if you have previously had a Caesarean section. You may, however, find it hard to get a booking, although it still remains your right. It is up to the health authority to make the best possible provision for your individual circumstances; this might include taking some blood for cross-matching in the event of your needing a blood transfusion, and making sure the midwife who attends you is experienced and has some back-up.

There are in fact a number of good reasons for having a baby at home after encountering difficulties with a previous birth, all of which contribute to reducing the chances of it happening again. Firstly, it is not your first baby and the vast majority of second or subsequent babies arrive far more easily than the first. You should feel completely relaxed in your surroundings; feel far freer to adopt any position, however unusual, that you instinctively feel will help the baby out; you will be able to eat and drink as you wish (see page 33 on how this can improve the outcome of labour); and you will be able to remain upright throughout labour, which is also influential in assisting the baby's passage. You will be far better able to respond intuitively to the message your body sends about the way to behave, and there is much less likely to be an atmosphere of controlled impatience and eagerness to get it all over and done with.

Because labour can only be accelerated in hospital, there is a far greater acceptance at home of it taking as long as it takes, and your midwife should be with you until the end. This is particularly important in the second stage, which in hospital is often limited to one hour for first time mothers and half an hour for women who have already had a child (although the NICE draft guidelines suggest women should be referred to a consultant after two hours and one hour respectively. After these intervals 'help' (usually ventouse or forceps) is often given automatically.

You will be more able to adopt the position of your choice to give birth if you are at home. This is of especial benefit to anyone who has experienced difficulty before, as a squatting position can widen the diameters of the outlet of the pelvis by as much as 5 cm, as well as being a position where gravity also helps the baby out.

Epidurals are not available at home, which can be an advantage as they are often responsible for a delay in the second stage when they can prevent reflex action of the muscles of the perineum from rotating the baby's head. They can also reduce the urge to push and are sometimes responsible for halting labour. Continuous electronic fetal monitoring is also unavailable, so that 'normal'

fetal distress is not detected and acted upon (see page 31 for expla-
nation). All these reasons are likely to ensure a good outcome in a
subsequent labour, but you can improve your chances still further
by consciously preparing for labour throughout pregnancy – see
the *How to help yourself* section on page 85.

For a more detailed analysis of previous problems see the following guide.

Ventouse and forceps

If you have had a baby delivered by ventouse (vacuum extraction)
or forceps, other than Keilland's rotation, you know that a baby can
come down through your pelvis. Ventouse or forceps are used for
a variety of reasons, including delay in the second stage, maternal
distress or exhaustion and fetal distress.

The delay can be due to the position of the baby's head, use of
an epidural and pushing while flat on your back. The baby's position
will not necessarily recur (see page 159 for ways of assisting posterior babies to shift); an epidural will not be repeated if you have
your baby at home; and you can make sure you don't push in a dis-
advantageous position again by practising squatting in pregnancy.

Maternal distress or exhaustion – another name for ketosis – is
unlikely to recur if you are eating and drinking properly and have
good support; the labour is likely to be quicker for a subsequent
child anyway. Some people think maternal distress also includes
such things as having heart disease or pre-eclampsia, when it is
thought better that you do not exert yourself by pushing. In these
cases it might be best to delay pushing as long as you possibly can
to minimise exertion. You might prefer to be in hospital, but this
should be your own decision. Marianne Monaco and Vicki Junor's
Home Birth Handbook[30] (now out of print) gives instances of
women with both these conditions who have given birth at home
satisfactorily.

Fetal distress is obviously specific to the individual baby. It can
be due to cord compression, placental insufficiency, maternal
hypotension (low blood pressure), epidural, maternal anxiety and
giving birth on your back (supine hypotension syndrome). Postmature babies may pass meconium (the greeny-black contents of
their bowels) into the amniotic fluid giving the appearance of being
in distress (see page 156). There is no reason why any of these things

should occur again, and some are clearly less likely to happen at home.

Caesarean section

There should be no automatic repeat Caesarean sections. In every case the need for this type of delivery should be assessed individually and in relation to the particular baby. The chances of having a vaginal birth following a Caesarean birth are good, although it will usually be described as a 'trial' of labour.

Such a birth is normally expected to take place in a consultant unit with facilities available for an emergency Caesarean section if necessary; this is because of the fear that your uterine scar may not stand up to the pressure of labour, and separate or rupture as a consequence. This happens only rarely – once in every 500 cases where the incision is of the lower-segment 'bikini line' kind. It is more common, 1-3 per cent, with classical up-and-down scar. In both cases it is more likely to occur when labour is artificially accelerated with Syntocinon.

If a scar does rupture, it is likely to do so at the end of pregnancy or in labour and it usually goes slowly. You might suspect it if you feel pain over the area of the scar which persists in between contractions, or have bleeding from the vagina. It might also be indicated by shock, swelling over the scar, a uterus which becomes rigid and does not contract, a rise in pulse rate or temperature or a fall in blood pressure. Clearly you should be admitted to hospital immediately in these circumstances. However, in most cases, separation is 'silent' so that neither the mother nor her attendants realise it until her uterus is checked following delivery, and it is then surgically repaired.

You are likely to face considerable opposition if you want to have a baby at home after a Caesarean section, although that experience may make you particularly keen to avoid a repetition. It has to be a confident and experienced midwife who will book you willingly, but it certainly has been done, even when there has not been a normal delivery in between. The general reluctance is a reflection of the obstetric practice in this country. In less developed countries home birth following Caesarean section is considered the norm, and it is generally trouble free if there is no evidence of gross disproportion of the pelvis.

In assessing whether the original reason for the operation is likely to be repeated, you need to bear in mind that although there will always appear to have been a convincing reason for operating, some operations are performed for reasons other than the health of mother or baby. These could include fear of litigation, lack of patience, theoretical but undemonstrated risk, and inexperience. Briefly, the reasons given could include:

- **Fetal distress.** This is particular to that baby and should not recur. If your baby had an initial Apgar score of 7 or above, he or she was not truly in distress. (The Apgar score is a means of rating a baby's condition at birth; it ranges from 1 to 10 and is done at one minute and again at five minute intervals until the baby scores 9.)
- **Failure to progress.** If your cervix does not dilate fully, the baby cannot be born and forceps cannot be used to help it out. This is a problem considered by many midwives to be associated with unhappiness in your surroundings, although it can also be mechanical, when the baby is too big for your pelvis. A home birth could be recommended if you remember feeling uneasy in hospital. If the reason was thought to be that the baby was too big for your pelvis, you should ask to have pelvimetry (an X-ray of your pelvis in various positions to assess its diameters) while you are not pregnant. This should give you a guide, although it is only a forecast. No one can be certain whether a baby will fit through a pelvis or not until labour. The baby has to be small if the transverse diameter at the outlet is 10 cm or less, but it is still not impossible. However if the same problem were to occur again at home, transfer would ultimately be inevitable.
- **Breech and other malpositions and malpresentations.** This would only be relevant if another baby was to adopt the same position, which can happen, although it need not.
- **Contracted pelvis.** This would remain the same. Again, it is worth having pelvimetry before you become pregnant again.
- **Herpes.** Some consultants consider this an automatic indication for Caesarean section. Others consider vaginal delivery is reasonable if there is no outbreak during the last four weeks of pregnancy, but this is controversial.
- **Failed ventouse or forceps.** You would have to know exactly

why instrumental delivery failed. Forceps should not have been used unless the baby's head was engaged in the pelvis and you were fully dilated. Pelvimetry might help here too. Remember that squatting can make all the difference between a normal or an operative delivery (see reference on page 81).

- **Pre-eclampsia.** This is much less likely in a subsequent pregnancy (4 per cent as opposed to 12 per cent), although if it does develop again and becomes severe, a repeat Caesarean section may well be necessary.
- **Placenta praevia.** This should not recur, but it would be useful to have a scan during late pregnancy to make sure.
- **Fibroids.** If untreated since the last pregnancy, fibroids might well be an indication for a repeat section if they obstruct the baby's way out, but they can degenerate without any treatment after pregnancy.

How you can help yourself

If you are planning a home birth after a previously difficult labour you will want to take definite steps to make labour easier this time. Getting the booking is probably the most important measure; you may find that once you are definitely booked, even if it is with difficulty, you feel a lot happier and more relaxed about the birth. In these circumstances it will be especially important to have a confident midwife. If you are thought to be at very high risk of developing complications for example with breech or twins, consider getting in touch with an independent midwife. Even if you do not employ her, you may get a more objective assessment of your situation. Ring her before you are pregnant or in early pregnancy if possible, and speak to more than one if you do not feel comfortable with the first.

Take the advice on page 114 about eating well and looking after yourself. Difficult labours are more common amongst poorly nourished women, and being fit can definitely help. There is increasing evidence to show the value of eating well in pregnancy. A cranial osteopath can treat a woman both pelvically and cranially to free the pelvis so that it works at its most efficient; this is done by making the connective tissue more elastic and thus making it less tight and restrictive. It is more effective than exercise alone, and can be strongly recommended for women with a history of previous problems. Ideally it should be started in early pregnancy. Taking raspberry leaf tea from 36 weeks of pregnancy onwards has been shown to make labour more efficient and specific treatment from a herbalist could help too.

You might also be helped by consulting a homeopath who could correct inbuilt weaknesses and who would be able to give you treatment to assist in labour. Some practitioners are willing to attend births, when they can give remedies as needed and help to ensure a good outcome.

It can make a great deal of difference to the mode of delivery if you practise squatting throughout pregnancy, and relax in positions which widen the pelvis to its greatest extent. If you are not used to it, you may not find squatting easy at first; however with persistence and daily practice you should be able to build up to around 15 minutes a day. The ideal position is on flat feet with your knees well apart and your back straight. If you find this difficult, start by supporting your back against a wall, and either wear shoes with heels or put a couple of books underneath your bottom.

WOMEN'S STORIES

"April brought the shock that we were expecting our fifth child. Our other children, then aged 16, 14, 12 and 6, were overjoyed, but it took me a long time to adjust, especially as I had returned to teaching and had just gained long overdue promotion.

"Our third and fourth children had been born at home (one in Yorkshire, the fourth in the house we live in at present in Northamptonshire, but on the Warwickshire border). There had been some caution from my GP and midwife when I asked to have the fourth at home, but eventually this went to plan, with a perfectly normal delivery that took 40 minutes from beginning to end. (We would never have made it to the hospital, which was over 18 miles away.)

"When I discovered number five was on the way and I was medically regarded as 'geriatric' (41 years!) I did not dare ask my GP for a home delivery – I knew he would not wish to take that responsibility and I did not wish to lose him as a GP as he is extremely good to us in every other way. However I became more and more anxious as time went on. Although most people

I saw at the hospital (a new unit had opened six miles away) were very pleasant, I took exception to the person in charge of the scanner; she was rude, wouldn't let fathers be present, noted that I had refused all tests for spina bifida, etc., and asked did I really want a 'defective child', saw that I had asked for a note 'No episiotomy unless absolutely necessary' on my card and demanded if I preferred to 'tear through to my anus' instead. When I realised that she also worked on the delivery ward from time to time I began to get very cold feet.

"The doctors that I saw, different ones on almost every occasion and never the specialist that I had been appointed to, were extremely polite and understanding, but here too I was assured that I would have to have the labour monitored because it was standard practice and safer for the baby.

"I asked if drips were used. I was told only if absolutely necessary, and yet I only spoke to one mother who had got away without one (her second baby, and she just refused in very strong tones). I knew I would refuse too – after all, if my fourth baby was born in 40 minutes from beginning to end, by how much would they wish to speed this one up? Again I was told episiotomies were not routine, but I could not find anyone who had avoided stitches. Eventually I became so depressed at the thought of going into hospital that I spoke to my local midwife. Fortunately she was pro home delivery. She gave me great hope and confidence. She wrote to the senior midwife of the county that we actually live in (the hospital I was booked into was in the adjacent county) and asked for her opinion on a home birth. My track record was excellent. Despite my 'great age' I was in very good health.

"The midwife put it to my GP that since baby four was born so quickly, perhaps it was a good idea to have a double delivery booked in case things happened faster than normal. Thus I was booked for home and hospital.

"Immediately I experienced a sense of calm and happiness, and the whole family was thrilled. I knew the baby would be born at home. My midwife was nothing less than wonderful.

"Seventeen days before D Day at 2.20 am my waters broke. We sent for our midwife. She arrived within 20 minutes, but I was not in labour. Our six-year-old woke up – I explained that the baby might be here by breakfast but that she was to go up to our elder daughter to sleep in her room (it was our personal preference that the older children would not be present at the birth).

"Breakfast time came. No baby. No labour. The midwife had gone back home at four o'clock saying she would return shortly after nine if we did not call sooner. All the children except the youngest went off to school by choice, armed with money for phone calls. Our little daughter went to my mother at the other end of the village.

"Our midwife explained that unfortunately if I didn't get into labour before 2.00 pm I would have to go in to hospital anyway. Would I agree to an enema? Yes. Ten past ten an enema was given. Ten-twenty the first pain was felt. Our midwife went to see another patient and gave us the phone number, promising to return in 40 minutes. Eleven-ten she returned. Eleven-twenty I was halfway to full dilation. Gas and air was most helpful by this time. Eleven thirty-five – full dilation. A phone call. My elder son from school. 'Is anything happening?' 'Yes.' My husband runs back upstairs. Eleven-forty Madeleine Sophie arrives – beautiful, the tiniest we've ever produced (6 lb 2 oz) but oh so fantastic.

"My husband phones mother and our little girl and they arrive within ten minutes (stage three not even over yet!). Our lovely midwife laughed – she had only managed to get one rubber glove on!

"So there we were, no postnatal depression, no stitches, no drips, no monitors or officious martinets, just another lovely child and lots of love."

Linda Hartley, *AIMS Journal*

"When when I was almost 40, I gave birth to my daughter Georgia at home. She was my fifth child and the first born at home. My obstetric history was mixed – first daughter born in hospital, straightforward, no drugs but a large (unnecessary?) episiotomy and lots of stitches. My second pregnancy ended in a miscarriage at 12 weeks and my third in a stillbirth at 40 weeks after a pregnancy, when my fears were expressed to many different antenatal staff but admission to hospital and weekly visits for almost the last three months failed to spot poor fetal growth – she weighed only 5 lb. By now a 'high-risk' mother,

I waited three years and then went on to have two sons just 14 months apart with no problems. For each of these deliveries I was assisted by excellent midwives and had no episiotomies or tears but I felt a growing conviction that hospital did not provide the right conditions for normal birth.

"When I became pregnant with Georgia I knew I wanted a home birth, but found it impossible to get agreement from my GP and the community midwives in the practice – they wouldn't even allow a domino. Finally I approached Jan Jennings, an independent midwife, booked with her and from then on I found I relaxed and my confidence grew.

"Labour began five days 'late', just as I was collecting my sons from school at 3.30. I had no 'show', no contractions and yet I was so sure that I telephoned my husband from school to ask him to come home. One of the boys went off happily with a friend, the other refused to leave me (it was good to be with him, chatting and reading until his sister arrived home). At home I phoned Jan and made the first of many pots of tea. By 4.30 when Jan arrived I was having irregular contractions and was only 2-3 cm dilated. Jan had called Nicky Leap and Katrina, a GP, and when they came at 5.00 I remember feeling a bit guilty at calling out all these people and not having anything more to justify it than an occasional, half-hearted contraction. So I made more tea, fed the children and went off for a bath. I found I didn't want to stay in very long but it relaxed me and when I dressed in a big, baggy shirt I'd worn often in pregnancy I felt comfortable too.

"After my bath I began pacing up and down the sitting room (where we had decided the baby would be born), backwards and forwards while the music played and I found myself retreating more and more inside myself, becoming less and less aware of everything and everyone around me. Contractions became stronger but not regular – two or three would come close together and then there would be a gap before the next group. When they were really painful I found leaning against Peter or Jan or the wall, with knees slightly bent, the most helpful, especially if my lower back was rubbed.

"At about 6.30 Nicky and Katrina left for a drink – I think we all felt that we might be in for a long night. However they had barely left the house when I had three huge contractions one after the other. I leaned hard against the wall, Jan rubbed my back and I found loud groaning a great help. I felt the baby move down and down. The contractions became long and strong with only a slight gap in between – they were difficult to manage and Jan suggested getting down on all fours, rocking and then looking at her, concentrating hard on blowing.

"There was a period of transition lasting about five minutes – I felt totally confused, unable to understand what I wanted to do. I sat down, stood up, knelt down, got up and turned round in circles. Then I found I knew exactly what I wanted and with Peter sitting down I squatted with my arms on his knees. I don't remember doing much pushing, it just happened by itself. The tape we had on finished playing, it was very quiet and, breathing gently, I felt the head emerge and out she slipped. It was 7.17. The cord was round her neck and as Jan removed it I reached down and scooped her up, warm and slippery, into my arms.

"We called the children in then (they had been watching TV) and they were quite amazed, fascinated by Georgia and only fleetingly interested in the still-attached cord. Five minutes later Nicky and Katrina arrived back. I put the baby to the breast where she latched on immediately, but after 20 minutes the placenta had not been delivered and we decided to cut the cord. Jan clamped it and I cut it. Third stage lasted some two hours although it seems the placenta detached quite quickly and there was little blood loss. I also found I didn't have 36 hours of sickness afterwards as I had previously when I'd had Syntometrine, and blood loss over the next few weeks seemed less.

"A few days later I saw the photos Sally Greenhill had taken of the birth. I found them amazing, firstly because I had been almost totally unaware of them being taken and also because they showed so clearly the emotions I remember experiencing and the pain, effort, enjoyment, exhilaration and joy of the whole event. Georgia is my last child. I'm glad she was born at home."

Christine Rodgers, *AIMS Journal*

'I really am a very small person, only 5 feet, with tiny hips and pelvis, and yet I gave birth very easily to an 8 lb 2 oz baby. I get extremely annoyed with consultants and midwives who make ridiculous statements that 'small' women have difficulty in giving birth. Given the opportunity and a favourable position for delivery I'm sure most women could deliver their babies successfully.

"We had no trouble whatsoever arranging a home birth. My doctor was surprised at such a request; his last home delivery was about 15 years ago. He was also a little anxious as my last baby was delivered by forceps after a very unfavourable and distressing labour, and an elective Caesarean was definitely on the cards for me if I had chosen to go to the hospital. I asked two consultants if I could be admitted to the GP unit for the delivery of my third baby – they both refused and announced a Caesarean birth was the only way out for my next baby.

"Well, after a very healthy and happy pregnancy I gave birth at home, safely and peacefully to a lovely boy in September. Even now, weeks later, I still feel dizzy with exhilaration. It was a lovely experience, so basic, yet so vitally important to fulfill. I enjoyed a very quick, exciting three-hour labour (my two previous hospital labours exceeded 24 hours). I had no drugs whatsoever, the thought of painkillers never crossed my mind. I was so happy and relaxed at home. I welcomed each contraction, knowing they brought the birth of my baby nearer. My husband applied firm pressure to my back while I stood and rubbed the tops of my legs. Honestly, this was sufficient to enable me to handle the contractions and I was so thrilled to be told I was already 7 cm dilated when the midwife arrived. I was expecting this unbearable pain to develop as I had experienced in hospital during my last labour, but it never arrived.

"My midwife was so sensitive, cheerful and supportive. She respected all my wishes and was happy to deliver my baby in a squatting position on the floor. After only a few pushes my baby was born and breastfed immediately. What a moment to treasure! To feel a warm, slippery, wide-eyed baby next to one's skin, whose senses are as alert as one's own is really what it is all about.

"The placenta was delivered in ten minutes without Syntometrine. My previous perineum scar tore a little and I had a few sutures, but they gave me no discomfort at all, unlike the extremely painful episiotomy I had had with the forceps delivery – it took seven months to heal.

"My home birth really was a perfect birth, so easy; it was

better than I ever imagined. It meant a great deal to me to deliver my baby myself, without drugs and interference. I felt in control the whole time. I firmly believe its success was due to the fact that my body was free to do its job properly, as nature intended. I just relaxed and savoured every moment. I envy midwives who can help a woman achieve this basic joyful function. I hope the choice of a home birth will always be available, and ideally I wish it was offered to all parents as a very attractive, safe place of birth. I shudder when I think I could have been robbed of this truly marvellous experience and suffered an elective Caesarean at the hands of a knife-happy consultant."

Linda Collier

"My first pregnancy was very straightforward and I expected it to be a textbook birth. Although I was having contractions from 40 weeks, I didn't go into labour and the midwife had me booked for induction for 12 days post-term as soon as I was 40 weeks pregnant. In hindsight we were like babes in the wood – we weren't given much advice about avoiding induction. I went in for induction and went into labour really quickly. I laboured for quite a while, lying down the whole time. After 12 hours I was begging for an epidural and my daughter was showing signs of distress. I got to 5 cm but no further, despite Syntocinon. They decided on a Caesarean section at 6.00 pm but because there were loads of us having c-sections that night, I didn't have her until 9.00. She was very alert and latched on immediately, but I was very shocked. I couldn't believe that I hadn't delivered her myself. Out of an antenatal group of five, four of us had c-sections in similar circumstances to mine – I felt that it was due to a cascade of intervention and lost a certain amount of faith in the NHS.

"When it came to having my second child, I wanted to avoid another major operation and to be physically fit enough to be able to pick up my daughter and show her affection afterwards. I also wanted to experience natural birth – I felt I had been robbed of that experience before. I thought the best way of giving myself a fighting chance of achieving this was by booking for a home birth and by getting a wise woman to help me.

"The specialist said that there was no way I could have a home birth – he said that I would be endangering my child and there was no way that he could support home birth, but the midwives were happy to book me and it seems that he was not aware of my booking.

"He was also not keen for my pregnancy to go past 40 weeks, but because of the c-section the only way of doing that was either by rupturing my membranes artificially or by elective Caesarean. Fortunately one of the other doctors was prepared to let it go to 42 weeks although not a day over, I was booked for an artificial rupture of membranes (ARM).

"I booked my doula fairly late – around 7 months. I felt that if she could help me achieve my aim it would be money well spent. I spoke to several but only one was free around the time I was due. She came to visit us for a face to face chat before we made a decision and I could see that we could work together. For the rest of the pregnancy I felt a lot more relaxed – I felt that Stacia knew a lot.

"This time I was determined to avoid induction and I was better informed. I tried herbs, hot curries, sex, walking long distances, self-hypnosis, pineapple and the midwives gave me a few cervical sweeps. It was a very exciting time – a real adventure. I felt quite bereft afterwards as I had been so well supported. I knew it wasn't far off – the house was full, Stacia was coming to the house and it was summertime. I had more herbs which seemed to work – the night before I was due for the ARM, the contractions I was getting increased. I called the midwife who came straight away. She did a sweep and then realised that she hadn't checked the baby's heartbeat first. When she did, she got my heartbeat by mistake and I think she panicked because it was much slower than it should have been, and said that we would have to go in. Although she checked again and found the baby's heartbeat and it was alright, she still wanted to go in. Part of me had been anxious about the home birth and thought 'Oh thank God'. After being transported by ambulance, we spent the night at the hospital – I was checked over, and then allowed to sleep until the morning. They wanted to do the ARM the following morning but it was delayed by other patients. After lunch I said 'Oh this really hurts!' – and the waters went naturally. Contractions were very strong and very painful – more so than with my first labour. I was determined to keep going, just have gas and air but I was falling asleep in the bath. The midwife thought that I was too relaxed and got me out.

"Meantime, I wasn't dilating – I was checked twice and was 3 cm each time. The consultant said that my cervix was badly swollen and that he didn't think it would go down to dilate. By 9 pm I was still 3 cm and I said 'Oh right – I will have an epidural'.

"Still there was no further dilation and Amit noticed on the monitor that the contractions were slowing down. Stacia left us on our own to discuss the situation – we decided we wanted the baby safe and well and he was delivered by caesarean. No one made any adverse comments about being booked for home, partly because we had kept very quiet about it. We only told a few select friends, not even my in-laws and most people didn't know that we had a birthing pool set up in our garage. People have strong feelings about home birth – I was quite shocked at how some people feel. We didn't want to listen to negativity, we wanted to be positive. We were happy with our decision and looking forward to it being a bit of a party.

"Talking about it afterwards, I felt that we made the right decisions. I am glad that we had the doula – I appreciated her information, her massage during labour – the fact that she gave my husband a role but took the burden of responsibility from him. She helped allay my worries – I wouldn't have been as happy without her. She took video clips and photos at the birth and was very good at doing things that will stay with us forever.

"I felt it was a great adventure, a much nicer and more exciting pregnancy than the first one, one in which I had really positive experiences. It opened my eyes to hypnotism and herbal remedies. I had a lot of support and felt from seven months onwards that I really could do it. Although it was not the outcome that I wanted I was grateful that I was able to have my baby safely and that the home birth option was well worth pursuing and very positive."

Lynn O'Connor

"I couldn't believe it when I reached the 11 March 2004 and I was still pregnant! I had endured the longest pregnancy in the history of the world, and patience being one of the qualities that I had in very short supply meant that reaching this due date still pregnant was an impossibility. I was beside myself and made sure that those around me knew my patience had reached its threshold!

"'Annie, when is this baby coming? How can I make it arrive, I've tried pineapple, curries, even a trip on the London Eye and nothing has happened – I can't bear to wait any longer, what can we do?' I wailed to my long suffering independent midwife Annie.

"Annie gave me a little bit of a talking to and pointed out, what were my options? Wait for nature to take its course, or go into hospital and be induced, at the same time saying goodbye to my home birth and a birth without intervention. After such a long, rollercoaster journey, to be here – still pregnant, healthy and finally being seen as low risk, I just needed to be patient.

"I totally trusted Annie. She was the only person on this long, long journey who had calmly and confidently kept all the options open and had never closed the door on this baby being born at home, despite my history.

"I had hired Annie in my previous pregnancy as I hated hospitals and knew I wanted a home birth. The hospital had told me they were short-staffed and often their homebirth service was suspended. I'd known I couldn't risk being made to go into hospital because of staff shortages, so at 18 weeks had taken the plunge and hired Annie and Tina from the South London Independent Midwives, to take on my care. Well, I would never have risked just turning up at a church hoping someone could marry us on my wedding day, so ensuring I had one-to-one care for the birth of my baby seemed the obvious thing to do.

"But when Annie had booked me in, we discovered that all was not well with that pregnancy. The rest of the world was getting ready for Christmas whilst we had dealt with the most devastating news – once again our hopes and dreams of creating our own family were shattered as we discovered we would lose that baby. At almost 20 weeks we had gone into hospital and I was induced. I gave birth to a tiny boy on 21 December 2002, with Annie and my husband at my side.

"When I had become pregnant again, I had been seen by the fetal medical specialist at the hospital. A home birth seemed an unlikely scenario. I thought I would limp to 28 weeks and need a Caesarean to rescue my baby from my useless body and its malfunctioning placentas.

"Occasionally I idealised about being able to have my baby at home, away from the clinical setting of the hospital I hated, but then my next appointment with the consultant would loom and I would feel once again that I was 'high risk' and lucky to still be pregnant!

"But at 36 weeks I had seen a different consultant, who told me that my pregnancy was looking good – I may once have been high risk, but now I was a normal, low risk, healthy pregnancy.

"'So does that mean I can have a home birth?' I had whispered, not daring to believe that he may say yes.

"'Can't see why not,' was his response. And so my home birth was back on the cards!

"'I had stayed calm, well relatively so I guess, and finally, five days past my due date, on the evening of 16 March 2004, at about 11.40 pm I felt my first contraction. I ran to the bathroom, my stomach churning.

"'Steve, I think that was a contraction,' I had nudged my sleeping husband. Very supportively he'd murmured 'well go back to sleep, it will be a long night, get some rest to keep your energy up'.

"'Go back to sleep? I'd like to see you sleep through one of those,' I muttered, but smiled, full of excitement. Finally this baby had decided to make an appearance.

The next two contractions came at 15 minute intervals, with me running to the bathroom.

About 12.30 am, the contractions were coming more quickly and strongly. I called to Steve as I knew I was about to be sick. He stumbled into the bathroom, and thrust the bucket in my direction just in time, as my body emptied itself of the previous few days of pineapple and curry!

By 1.10 am, the contractions were coming harder and faster and I was being sick at the beginning, middle and end of each one or so it seemed.

"'Call Annie', I breathed to Steve, 'I need her now'. I could sense that I was beginning to lose control and knew I needed to give myself over to the process, leave the rational thoughts to someone else and just go with the labour.

"'Hmm I'm not sure,' came his reply to my complete astonishment – 'I think it may have been something we ate – I've got a slightly uncomfortable tummy too, but I had some Rennies and they helped – why don't you try having one.'

"'Oh God,' I moaned puffing between contractions. 'A Rennie won't do it, I'm having a baby,' I groaned back at him. 'Call Annie now'.

"Something in the tone of my voice – or maybe by just trying to look me in the eye and realising I was locked into a different place, sent him looking for the phone.

"'Hi there Annie, sorry to disturb you so late, but Roz has told me to call you, she thinks she's in labour and is quite keen for you to come over . . . ' I could hear him in the background, politely talking to Annie.

"Thankfully Annie could hear me, groaning, puffing and vomiting in the background and told Steve she was on her way.

"She arrived about 1.50 am. I remember the sense of relief flooding through me when she came into the bathroom. Confidence and calm reigned once again!

"In between the fast and furious contractions Annie made sure I was OK, and checked out whether I wanted to stay in the bathroom or move elsewhere. Having previously envisaged that I would romantically give birth in the lounge, with an open fire, burning essential oils of rose and jasmine, when it came to it, here I was, in the bathroom, the smallest room possible and I didn't want to move.

"My labour was, I guess, relatively quick – although at times it felt endless. Tina must have arrived at some point but I have no recollection of what time, but had a vague recollection of the bathroom getting more crowded.

"The second stage seemed to take forever, with Steve holding my hands and bracing so I could rise up and down to try and encourage our baby on his way.

"Finally I remember Annie asking me if I wanted to touch the baby's head – I declined, petrified that I might inadvertently push my baby's head back inside me. But another push and at 5.59 am I felt our baby arrive.

"I looked down, and saw these two huge, bright, shiny eyes, darting about, not missing a thing, taking it all in.

"'Oh my goodness, look, look at our baby . . . ' I inadvertently moved the umbilical cord and spotted his sex, 'it's a boy, a beautiful wonderful baby boy, he looks just like you, Steve.' I sobbed, elated and overcome with the joy and wonder of it all.

"Both Steve and Annie had wet eyes – Tina was hidden from view as our bathroom wasn't really big enough for four adults, a birth ball and a new baby! Finally he was here, this tiny little baby, who we had waited for so long, arriving in the most incredible way. He was our miracle baby – not least because he arrived having the cord wrapped twice around his neck and with a double knot in it! (Thank you to whoever made sure he made it!)

"I was just bursting: with pride, with love, with delight! I offered him my breast, but he was more interested in eye contact – watching us all, shiny eyed, bright, a huge personality. His placenta took only minutes before it dropped away naturally, and then still marvelling at the perfectness of our son, we cut his extremely long cord and he was weighed.

"Steve ran the bath for me and I clambered in – I remember being so grateful to be here in my own bath, my own home, nothing antiseptic or medical, just here with my husband and new son. I wallowed in my bath, enjoying both a cup of tea and a glass of champagne, revelling in the joy of spending the first few magical moments together as a family in our own home.

"Then, Eddie and I were wrapped into one of our own, huge soft towels and gently dried, lovingly by my dearest husband. We tiptoed up the hallway carrying our precious Eddie, and climbed into our own, comfortable bed, in our bedroom. We were tucked up by Annie and Tina and left to sleep. Sleep, my dear husband and the miniature version of him lying between us did, whilst I marvelled at the wonder of nature, the happiest, hormonally high girl in the whole world.

"My home birth is still to this day one of the things I am most proud of – I see it as an achievement way above any career successes. I had my baby at home, after a roller coaster pregnancy. I did that – I gave birth to my little boy, in the most natural place, in the home where he was conceived."

Roz Collins

8   complications of pregnancy

This chapter covers complications of pregnancy, and the question of whether such complications – either past or present – mean that you should accept a hospital delivery. The question has to be dealt with because the threat of complications is sometimes used by health professionals to persuade you to change your booking. This may either be because they are opposed to home birth or very nervous about it. The result is that you have to examine any claim of this kind so you are able to assure yourself of its validity.

It can be very hard to be objective about such matters. If a home birth is being denied you because of some specific factor relating to you or your baby, it is difficult to assess the situation unemotionally and work out really what is best. This is because the nature of motherhood means that women will always put their babies' well-being before that of their own, and any suggestion that they are putting their child at risk will affect them powerfully. So, even if you suspect the motives of your advisors, it can still be very difficult to defy them; you are always left with the nagging fear that they might be right, even when intellectually you are sure that they are not. Of course this instinct is well appreciated by those used to dealing with pregnant women, and it is successfully exploited as a means of coercion.

In some instances of complications there will be no doubt at all in your mind that you need hospital facilities. In fact you may even be keener to get there than your midwife. In others, though, it may be a lot less clearcut. The matter in question may be one of degree or opinion – some midwives would transfer you, others would not (and it is clear that there are regional variations, see page 153). Remember that Marjorie Tew found that hospital was only of benefit to women at very high risk of complications and that even then the risk was equal to being delivered elsewhere, that babies were not at increased risk because they were not being born in a consultant unit. Other cases may be even more nebulous. For example it is not easy for a woman to check her blood pressure for herself, and even with genuinely raised blood pressure it is quite usual to feel well. If your doctor tells you it is high, is it strategic or authentic, and even if it is truly raised would you be better off in hospital? Sadly there are examples of this sort of coercion by complication, making it vital for you to be convinced that something really is amiss before changing your booking. Being left with lingering doubts can be damaging and will detract from your whole-hearted enjoyment of your baby.

The following is a list of the more common types of complication, with suggestions as to how to assess their gravity and suggestions as to remedies. It includes problems arising in a current pregnancy.

However, I have not dealt with existing conditions such as diabetes, kidney and heart disease, essential hypertension and thyroid problems, which are hard to generalise about. It is best to find out as much as you can about the likely course of labour and make up your own mind. You will need support for a decision to have a baby at home if you have such a complaint and it might well be worth contacting an independent midwife.

PRE-ECLAMPSIA AND ECLAMPSIA

Eclampsia, and its forerunner pre-eclampsia (toxaemia of pregnancy, or pregnancy-induced hypertension), is a disease unique to pregnancy. Its cause is not fully understood, although it is thought it may be immunological. If untreated it causes severe convulsions in the mother, and can lead to the death of the mother and fetus. Its existence is the reason why blood pressure testing plays such a large part of antenatal care.

Pre-eclampsia consists of three main symptoms: a large rise in blood pressure; a large weight gain due to fluid retention; and protein in the urine due to the breakdown of kidney tissue. It is more common in first pregnancies (12 per cent) than in subsequent ones (4 per cent). It is a condition which can come on quite suddenly, so that if you have one or more of the following pre-eclamptic signs you should get medical aid straight away:

- Severe headaches, unrelieved by taking pain killers.

- Visual disturbances, like seeing flashing lights.
- Abdominal pain.
- Considerable swelling of the body.

However your blood pressure can be raised without the accompanying signs. It starts to cause concern when the diastolic pressure (the lower figure shown in your notes, e.g. 120/70) is raised by more than 20 points over what is normal for you in pregnancy. The diastolic pressure indicates the pressure in your arteries when the heart is at rest. Normal pregnant blood pressure ranges between 90/50 and 140/90. If your blood pressure reaches 140/90 or more you will normally be expected to rest, and you will have it checked more frequently. Raised blood pressure is of concern because, as well as the risk of your developing pre-eclampsia, it can mean that there is a reduction in the supply of blood and oxygen to the baby.

Blood pressure is difficult to check yourself, but it is possible to get an independent opinion. Any trained alternative practitioner should be able to take blood pressure and also give you some treatment to reduce it – it might be helpful to consult a herbalist or homeopath. You can also buy kits designed for do-it-yourself blood pressure testing or get it checked at a chemists.

How you can help yourself

The first treatment for raised blood pressure is rest. Although it is possible that exercise may help by forcing blood through the vessels, this is not advocated conventionally and you will be expected to rest much more, perhaps all day. You can help by lying on your left-hand side, because this increases the flow of blood to the placenta. You should make sure that you are eating frequently and well, including plenty of protein in your diet. Controversy rages about the place of salt in your diet, but it seems sensible to have a moderate amount.

Other suggestions include taking a vitamin B-complex supplement that includes 50 mg of vitamin B6 daily, and six dolomite tablets to increase magnesium and calcium intake. Garlic, either raw or in the form of garlic perles (two to ten daily), should help and cayenne pepper taken in yoghurt or orange juice ($\frac{1}{4}$-1 teaspoonful three times a day) can be useful in normalising blood pressure. Also try dandelion leaves, either raw or cooked, and take at least two cups of dandelion tea per day. Lime blossom tea can help as well.

Another practical suggestion is to see if you can have your blood pressure checked by a community midwife whilst you are at home. Of course this will not be satisfactory if you do not feel that you are able to trust your midwives, but it can be very helpful if you are one of the people affected by 'white coat hypertension' – this occurs when your blood pressure is raised in clinic or hospital but is otherwise normal. It can be useful to ask to have your blood pressure checked again at the end of your visit if it has been high at the start. Tension and the energy expended in getting to your antenatal appointment, especially if you already have children, is traditionally only expected to affect the systolic pressure (the pressure generated by your heart as it pumps); however experienced midwives recognise that the anxiety that can be generated by these appointments can affect both systolic and diastolic readings.

However, if your blood pressure reaches a level of 150/100 you are strongly recommended to go into hospital because of the serious risk to life for you and your baby. If it is not reduced by bed rest, and the baby is close to term, you will probably have labour induced or be delivered by Caesarean section. Raised blood pressure earlier in pregnancy may be treated by drugs.

BLEEDING

Bleeding in pregnancy is not normal but is not uncommon. Technically such bleeding falls into two categories: bleeding before 28 weeks due to various causes, including threatened or complete miscarriage; and bleeding after 28 weeks, which is known as antepartum haemorrhage and includes bleeding at the start of labour. Bleeding is always regarded seriously, with the added anxiety for a woman wanting to have her baby at home as to whether reporting a bleed will result in her home booking being revoked. She may also feel that, if it is inevitable that she miscarries, she would prefer to do so at home as well. It is therefore important to describe the types of bleeding and their possible causes and discuss when it may be essential to seek hospital treatment.

Bleeding before 28 weeks

There are several causes of bleeding before 28 weeks. It is fairly common to experience bleeding at the time of a missed period at 4, 8 and 12 weeks of pregnancy. This occurs when the levels of pregnancy hormones are insufficiently high to suppress menstrual bleeding completely. It should be much less than a normal period and cease around the 14-week stage, when the placenta takes over hormone production from the corpus luteum (a yellow body which grows on the ovary at the site of the ruptured egg follicle and initially sustains the pregnancy).

Bleeding can also be due to polyps on the cervix – small, benign growths which, like cervical erosions, can cause bleeding after intercourse. They may be seen with the aid of a speculum and are not serious.

Ectopic pregnancy is a less common, but potentially very serious, cause of bleeding in early pregnancy. It is caused by the pregnancy becoming established in some part of the reproductive system other than the uterus – frequently the Fallopian tube. Bleeding starts between 6 and 12 weeks, most often from eight weeks onwards. It is sometimes accompanied by one-sided abdominal pain and can be confused with appendicitis. Eventually the Fallopian tube ruptures, causing considerable pain and shock and further bleeding, both internally and from the vagina. Ectopic pregnancy constitutes a surgical emergency, surgery being essential to remove the embryo and remove or repair the tube.

Very rarely bleeding is caused by a hydatidiform mole. This is a pregnancy where there is an abnormal development of the placenta and no fetus. Grape-like vesicles are passed and bleeding is likely to be accompanied by acute nausea and vomiting.

The major cause of early pregnancy bleeding, though, is due to miscarriage. This is said to be 'threatened' when bleeding, and sometimes pain, is present but contractions do not open the cervix. If the cervix opens, miscarriage is said to be 'inevitable'. The bleeding will increase and the contractions expel the fetus – the miscarriage is then said to be complete; or the bleeding will continue, sometimes very severely, but the contents of the uterus are not fully expelled – the miscarriage is then said to be incomplete.

Incomplete miscarriages, and often complete ones too, are treated in hospital. If the bleeding is severe, an injection of ergometrine is given into the thigh; as with postpartum bleeding (page 189), this works by contracting the uterus down tightly so that the site of bleeding is reduced. Once the bleeding has decreased, preparation is made for dilation and curettage (D and C, also known as ERPC — evacuation of retained products of conception) of the uterus under general anaesthetic. This involves gentle dilation of the cervix and scraping of the uterine wall to detach and remove any fetal or placental tissue that may remain. This can be important if the miscarriage is not complete because tissue that is not removed can lead to continued bleeding and possible infection.

Missed abortion

This is where the fetus dies but is not expelled. You may suspect it if you have a brown discharge and no longer feel pregnant.

Antepartum bleeding

This is bleeding from the vagina before delivery; a certain amount of bleeding can be expected at the start of labour, when the mucus plug that fills the cervix throughout pregnancy is detached by the dilation of the cervix in early labour. Blood is often mixed with the mucus but it should not be excessive in amount and will probably not soak through a pad.

More serious causes of bleeding in this period can be due to blood loss from the placenta, either because it is separating prematurely, as in *placenta abruptio*, or because it has implanted in such a position as to block the opening to the cervix, called *placenta praevia*.

With *placenta abruptio* the bleeding is combined with a severe pain in the abdomen. This is caused by the placenta peeling away from the wall of the uterus, and it can give rise to a continuous pain which does not come and go in waves like contractions. Blood loss may be vaginal or it may be contained within the uterus and so not be visible. The abdomen itself is likely to be, and stay, rock-hard and the mother will be shocked (see page 154). In these circumstances the baby may need to be delivered by Caesarean section as a matter of urgency.

There are degrees of *placenta praevia*, depending on where the placenta implants and how much of it is over the cervix. It might be suspected when there is bright red, painless bleeding in later pregnancy, or when a baby persistently lies across the abdomen and never becomes either head or bottom down. An abnormally placed placenta can be detected by ultrasound. A placenta that does not quite reach the cervix, or just covers the edge, may mean you can be delivered vaginally, although perhaps it should be in hospital, in case bleeding is excessive. Caesarean section is necessary when the placenta covers more of the cervix or blocks it completely.

What you can do

Bleeding in pregnancy is always worrying. The conventional advice to women on discovering that they are bleeding is to call a doctor and immediately go to bed, or, if the bleeding is heavy, to call an ambulance. However, there are various reasons why some women prefer not to do this.

Firstly, for some women, especially those for whom it is not their first pregnancy, bleeding seems to be relatively normal. For example a small survey of women suffering from endometriosis, a common condition where uterine tissue grows outside the uterus, found that as many as 50 per cent experienced bleeding in pregnancy, sometimes on and off throughout the pregnancy. Although they may not feel happy about it, they may feel that they can cope with it and would rather manage at home than be hospitalised.

Other women feel that, even if they are miscarrying, they would rather miscarry in the comfort of their own home, for many of the same reasons that they were choosing to have their babies at home. Women who have previously had hospital treatment for miscarriage often opt to stay at home if it happens again. This is not least because of the insensitivity with which miscarriage is sometimes treated by hospital staff.

The other point about consulting a doctor for lesser degrees of bleeding is that, apart from recommending bed rest, there is very little in the way of treatment. Moreover there is often an assumption that once you have been admitted to hospital at any point during the course of pregnancy, the delivery is automatically going to take place there. It is a great pity if you feel that you cannot admit to having problems because it will mean you are now no longer able to choose the place of delivery (although, of course, you still have the right to insist). However, if women are under pressure to have a hospital birth, reporting mild bleeding, for example, can feel like throwing in the towel completely. Feeling like this can make you very isolated, so you may be helped by some guidelines on bleeding in pregnancy. Your instinct for self-preservation is unlikely to let you down by failing to make you aware when it is really essential to get medical help.

You should contact a doctor or midwife if:

- You would feel happier in hospital.
- Bleeding is severe and/or accompanied by pain, particularly one-sided pain in the early weeks, or a rigid abdomen in later weeks.
- You have painless, bright red bleeding in the later weeks and you have not had a scan to show placental position.

What they can do:

- Advise bed rest. You may get more real rest in hospital depending on your circumstances, but you will probably feel happier at home.
- Do an ultrasonic scan to establish where the placenta is and if the fetus is alive.
- If miscarriage has become inevitable, give ergometrine to stop severe bleeding and perform an ERPC under general anaesthetic.
- Induce labour if the baby has died but labour has not started naturally.

But there are things you can do to help yourself:

- Go to bed and rest, lying on your left side to increase the blood flow to the placenta. Make sure that you are eating well, and avoid anything containing caffeine (coffee, chocolate, cola), alcohol and smoking. Accept as much help as possible, particularly if you feel you cannot rest. Rest has not been proved to prevent miscarriage, and plenty of women who have experienced bleeding in pregnancy have given birth to healthy babies. However, you may feel happier if you do rest, and perhaps have the consolation that you did all you could, should you go on to lose the baby.

- Consider alternative remedies. An alternative practitioner such as an acupuncturist, herbalist or homeopath may very well be able to offer you treatment to stop the bleeding, whatever the cause. Alternative medicine has a far greater scope than Western medicine and has specific remedies for problems such as this, where there is no orthodox equivalent. An acupuncturist would treat you twice within 24-36 hours and perhaps give you moxa (a slow burning herb) to use at home to warm specific acupuncture points. He or she might also advise you about diet and rest. This treatment would be effective unless the baby was damaged, in which case the miscarriage would continue. Herbalists or homeopaths would provide herbs or pills specifically for you and the cause of your bleeding.
- Try increasing your vitamin intake. The following have been suggested as helpful in stemming bleeding in pregnancy:
    Vitamin E – up to 2,000 iu daily.
    Zinc – 25 mg daily.
    Manganese chloride or amino-chelate – 10-20 mg daily.
    Essential fatty acids – 1-4 g evening primrose oil daily.
- If you cannot reach an alternative practitioner, you might want to try taking any of the following herbal remedies:
    False unicorn root (Helonias or Chamaelirum luteum) – 15 g to a pint (600 ml) of water, boiled and then simmered gently for 15 minutes. Drink freely throughout the day. Alternatively try 20-30 drops of the tincture, three times a day.
    Wild yam root – take 50-120 ml of decoction, prepared in the same way as the False Unicorn root, every half hour.
    You could also try a 50:50 combination of the tinctures of Chamaelirium luteum and Viburnum prunifolium. Take 10-20 drops in a little cold water every 15-60 minutes until the bleeding stops, gradually reducing to 20 drops each morning until 22 weeks.
- Avoid intercourse for two weeks after the bleeding has ceased. If the bleeding followed intercourse, it may have been caused by cervical polyps or erosions. It can be helpful to ask if these appear to be present if you have a routine vaginal examination.

If the bleeding continues

The bleeding will continue and increase in intensity if a threatened miscarriage becomes inevitable. The exception to this may be in the case of missed abortion, where the only sign that the fetus is dead may be intermittent dark brown discharge and a decrease in the feeling of being pregnant. Signs of miscarriage are:

- **The os, the opening in the cervix, opens.** You should not try and feel for this yourself as there is a risk of introducing infection, and manual stimulation of the cervix may stimulate prostaglandins and initiate contractions (as in a cervical sweep at full-term). It is for these reasons that any medical examination of your cervix should be done by means of a speculum alone.
- **Pain.** It is rare for women not to experience pain with a miscarriage, although it may vary in type. Continuous pain, cramps, period-type pains and backache have all been reported.
- **Bleeding.** Some fetuses are miscarried with relatively little bleeding but in most cases quite a lot of blood will be lost. Obviously, it is very important to be sure that you do not risk losing too much blood, and it can be difficult to judge how much you are losing. You should get help if you also feel faint, cold, clammy or you have ringing in your ears or feel very thirsty. Other signs of excessive blood loss, and therefore shock, are sweating, gasping for air or feeling breathless, seeing spots before the eyes or having blurred vision and generally feeling weak. You are likely to feel great sadness although your immediate concern is, quite rightly, likely to be for your own life.

It can be very difficult to know if you have actually miscarried, particularly if it is quite early in the pregnancy or if you have passed large clots but are not sure if you have lost the fetus as well. It is possible to bleed quite heavily and yet go on to give birth to a healthy baby.

You can be certain that you have had a complete miscarriage if the whole sac of membranes is delivered intact. In this case they will look like a big wobbly ball, with the fetus visible in the middle.

The outside of the membranes will be bloody where the placenta is attached to it. It will also be clear that you have miscarried if you find the fetus amongst the blood clots and placental tissue. In this case, you may not be able to tell if any tissue has been retained and you may need an ERPC. Complete miscarriage will be followed by a decrease in bleeding, an end to the pain (although miscarriages after 20 weeks may be followed by after-pains) and a definite sensation of having passed something. Your doctor may be able to tell whether the miscarriage has been complete if he or she is able to examine everything that has come away. It is for this reason that women are traditionally urged to keep what are known medically as 'the products of conception'. However, if you do miscarry and do not want to involve a doctor, it is possible for you to dispose of the baby as you wish, because there are ways of working out whether you need medical help (see below).

Incomplete miscarriage, when only part of the fetus or tissue has been expelled, is potentially more dangerous because it can lead to severe bleeding and shock. In this case bleeding will not stop, the pain does not cease and you definitely need an ERPC.

Retained tissue following miscarriage will mean that the bleeding will not gradually cease. It may continue to be bright red and you might go on passing clots. This is more common if you have not had an ERPC, although it seems likely that the operation is frequently performed when it is not essential (the medical dictum being 'If in doubt scrape it out').

Retained tissue may result in infection, although again this is quite possible following hospital treatment. This will result in: an evil-smelling discharge which may contain pus (and blood); abdominal pain of an intermittent nature; raised temperature; flu-like symptoms; and possibly itching and irritation of the vagina. It is very important to get it promptly treated with antibiotics as it can lead to sterility otherwise.

If you are rhesus negative and the baby's father is rhesus positive, it is important to get an anti-D injection within 72 hours of birth, miscarriage or even a threatened miscarriage so that you do not run the risk of developing antibodies to rhesus positive blood which might harm subsequent children.

An acupuncturist can treat you for retained tissue. Herbalists can treat infection and homeopathy can treat your emotions. A practitioner using Bach flower remedies might be able to help your feelings of loss and sadness. Cranial osteopathy (from an osteopath trained in working through your head) and herbs can help you recover from a general anaesthetic much more rapidly. If you lose much blood you could take Floradix, a herbal iron preparation available from healthfood shops, to prevent anaemia making you feel weak and unable to cope. NDS Plus contains iron and other ingredients including folic acid in an easily absorbed form (see **www.ndshealthcare.com**).

ABNORMALITY DETECTED IN PREGNANCY

This depends on whether or not you elect to have some of the more sophisticated antenatal screening tests, as they are generally the only way a definitive diagnosis of fetal abnormality can be made before birth. Choosing to have such screening can be a difficult decision. This is not only because if you are choosing a home birth you may well dislike the high-tech aspects of conventional hospital antenatal care, but also because any visit to a hospital (and these tests are only available in hospital) may provide an opportunity for hospital staff to put pressure on you to change your mind about your place of delivery. Moreover there are proven risks associated with tests such as amniocentesis, so that you have to be sure that the benefits outweigh the disadvantages.

If abnormality is detected you will have even harder decisions to make. You will have to decide if the abnormality is sufficiently serious to warrant termination of the pregnancy. You will want to know whether the diagnosis is absolutely certain, whether anything can be done to remedy the situation, and whether the baby is likely to live. If the condition is not sufficiently severe to consider termination or you would not consider termination in any case (the tests should not be conditional on accepting termination in the case of abnormality), you will have to think again about where to have the baby. Depending on the nature of the problem, you might want to have the baby in hospital with specialist resuscitation facilities. On the other hand you might find it best to have the baby at home where the opportunity for 'officiously striving to keep alive' are limited, and it is easier to let nature take its course. If the condition is incompatible with life you might rather your baby spent its short life in its own home rather than in a hospital special care unit. The balance of power in these sorts of situations are very different, depending on the place of delivery. It is far more difficult, if not impossible, to prevent a sick baby receiving treatment with which you do not agree if it is under hospital care than if it is in your own home.

For all these, and other, reasons you might want to think carefully before accepting ultrasound, amniocentesis or chorionic villus sampling.

Ultrasound

Ultrasonagraphy provides a picture of a fetus by means of bouncing high-frequency sound waves off the baby. It is useful for dating the pregnancy, checking for major abnormalities, to see if there is more than one baby, locating the placenta and assessing the cause in cases of bleeding in pregnancy. It is routine in many hospitals at around 16 weeks of pregnancy, and you may be under pressure to accept a scan even if you are having your baby at home.

The actual procedure involves lying on your back on a narrow trolley while a blunt probe is scanned across your abdomen, which is lubricated with conductive gel. A sometimes blurred picture is built up on a nearby screen. It is possible to freeze the picture so that specific measurements of the baby can be made to assess the gestational age.

You might prefer not to have a routine scan if you are sure of your dates and would prefer not to know if the baby had an abnormality, or would not choose termination if it had. If you are having more than one baby the fact is almost certain to be detected by abdominal palpation at a later stage, but you might opt for a scan if you felt there was reason to suspect a multiple birth. This might be because you put on an unusual amount of weight, your girth was bigger than that of other women at the same stage of pregnancy, you felt a lot of movement, or were excessively nauseous or experienced a lot of vomiting. Some mothers expecting more than one baby find they get extra tired. It is important to know if you are having twins if you want a home birth.

The benefits of ultrasound can be considerable, however it may be too early to be certain that it is completely harmless. After all, X-raying unborn children was initially thought to be harmless, and subsequently turned out to cause malignancies in childhood. Questions are starting to be raised about its safety; if you have any doubts about it, look at the article by Marsden Wagner on ultra-sound published in *Midwifery Today* (**www.midwiferytoday.com**).

AIMS can supply you with a sheet for your baby's ultrasound record to be filled in by the operator. See **www.aims.org.uk** for information about how to obtain one.

Although undoubtedly very valuable in situations where there is some reason to be concerned about the pregnancy, there are instances where the routine use of ultrasound gives rise to anxiety and its accuracy is in question. Its value as a diagnostic tool is dependent on the skill of the operator: it is possible for major abnormalities such as exomphalos (where the gut develops outside the abdomen) to go undetected by relatively unskilled operators; its accuracy for dating and detecting babies that are not growing well are also questionable; and it may also pick up abnormalities that appear to be present in pregnancy but which are not there at birth. These situations are responsible for considerable distress and may have a lasting effect on a mother's relationship with her child; clearly this cannot arise if you do not have ultrasound.

Amniocentesis

This is a non-routine test used to investigate the baby's chromo-some make-up and can be used to determine its sex and some physical abnormalities, such as neural tube defects like spina bifida and anencephaly. It can also detect some enzyme disorders such as phenylketonuria and Tay Sachs disease. It might be used if you have a higher than average chance of having an abnormal baby, perhaps because of your age; the chances of having a baby with Down's syn-drome or other chromosome abnormality increases with your age so that it rises from 1 in 1,923 at the age of 20 to 1 in 109 when you are 40.

Amniocentesis on the basis of maternal age is usually offered at some point between the ages of 35 and 40, depending on the pol-icy of the health authority. It is offered to all women over 40 and also to all those who already have an affected child, those who are known to be carriers of sex-linked diseases such as haemophilia, those with a family history of chromosome abnormalities and those whose alphafetoprotein test results suggest that there may be a problem with the baby.

The test is not usually performed until 16 weeks of pregnancy. It involves drawing off 20 ml of amniotic fluid and then culturing the fetal cells within that fluid for two and a half weeks. The chromosomes are then photographed and counted. This means that you do not get the results for at least three weeks so that you may be 19 weeks pregnant before you know the outcome. It is important to know that 5 per cent of cultures fail to grow and have to be repeated, there is a 0.5 per cent risk of an error in the result and a slight risk of introducing infection into the uterus or of the baby being injured by the needle, and there is a 1 per cent chance that the procedure will cause a miscarriage. It is also possible that the removal of amniotic fluid will cause some compression of the fetus. Amniocentesis is also said to increase the chance of placental abruption and breathing difficulties in the new-born baby. The authors who make this last claim also state that for reasons which are not understood, there is a 30 per cent higher incidence of chromosomal abnormality at amniocentesis than at birth, which poses the disturbing question of whether terminations for abnormality are performed needlessly.[31]

Amniocentesis may be painful and you should rest for a minimum of 24 hours afterwards to reduce the chance of it starting contractions.

Choronic villus sampling (CVS)

This is done at an earlier stage of pregnancy than amniocentesis and is not yet available everywhere. Like amniocentesis, it is performed in hospital and involves the use of ultrasound. The test is done by removing a few of the villi from the developing fetal placenta from the outside of the developing gestational sac. These villi, which surround the sac in the early weeks, disappear by about 13 weeks, leaving only the placenta.

Once the villi are removed they can be tested directly for sex and some blood, chromosome and metabolic disorders. Because cells do not have to be grown in a culture the results are available much sooner, usually in about five days. The test is relatively painless, although the cervix has to be held steady and there may consequently be some bleeding. You will be advised to avoid intercourse and vigorous exercise for five days afterwards. The disadvantages are that having CVS increases your chance of miscarrying by 2 per cent, and again there can be both false positive and negative results. It is not able to show up neural tube defects, so that amnio-centesis is still necessary if such problems are to be excluded with certainty. CVS is beginning to fall from favour as a method of early genetic screening, following the discovery that a few babies tested in this way had mild limb abnormalities. More details about this and other tests from the Genetic Interest Group, **www.gig.org.uk**.

Nuchal fold testing

A form of testing for Down's syndrome which involves examining the neck area of babies via ultrasound between 11-13 weeks of pregnancy. It may be combined with blood testing to give you an estimated individual risk ratio.

What to do

Fortunately the question of what to do following a diagnosis of abnormality in pregnancy arises only rarely. However it is an issue of such complexity that it is not possible to offer any guidelines. You might want to contact a self-help group like Antenatal Results and Choices (see **www.arc-uk.org**) for further information and advice.

Minimising the risk

There are ways in which you can minimise the chance of having a baby with problems, some of which involve taking steps before you become pregnant. This would obviously be worth considering if you have already had an affected child or if you have a family history that suggests your baby might be at risk. In these circumstances it would be a good idea to seek genetic counselling, which can be arranged through your GP.

- Make sure that you are eating well. This is generally held to mean cutting out, or at least down on, refined foods such as biscuits, cakes, sweets, high-fat foods like chips, and foods that contain large amounts of sugar, additives and artificial colourings. Eat fresh rather than manufactured foods, concentrating on meat, fish, eggs, cheese, wholegrains, pulses, nuts, fruit and vegetables.

- If you are a vegetarian make sure that you are taking a vitamin B12 supplement.
- Take a broad spectrum multivitamin and mineral supplement which includes 0.4 mg of folic acid. Folic acid should be included in a woman's diet from the time she starts trying to conceive until at least 28 days of pregnancy (government guidelines suggest you should take it up until 12 weeks). This has been shown to reduce the incidence of neural tube defects in babies born to mothers who have already had one affected baby.
- Take vitamin E, 200-400 iu daily (it has been suggested that this amount be increased to 500-15,000 iu daily in women who have already had a child with an abnormality).
- Get your partner to start taking the multivitamin at least three months before a planned conception. There are specific pre-conception formulas for both men and women available.
- Get your blood tested before pregnancy to make sure that you are immune to rubella. Women who have been pregnant before will have had their blood tested already and will have been offered immunisation after birth if they were not immune.
- Both of you should take 25-50 mg elemental zinc daily.
- Try to cut out smoking and alcohol consumption. Substitute herbal or fruit teas for coffee and ordinary tea. Even one cup of coffee a day has been shown to reduce fertility and there is some question about whether caffeine is responsible for an increase in birth defects.
- Drink plenty of spring water.
- Avoid eating cheese made from unpasteurised milk, soft cheeses, cook-chill foods, manufactured paté and ready-prepared salads off the supermarket shelf as these can carry listeria bacteria which can be fatal in the unborn child.
- Be very careful about washing your hands after handling animals, and try to avoid handling cat litter trays. If unavoidable wear rubber gloves and use boiling water.
- Do not eat raw or undercooked meat. Wash your hands thoroughly after preparing meat.
- Stop any non-essential drugs and discuss the use of essential drugs with your GP or consultant.

MALPOSITION

A baby's position in the uterus generally becomes fixed at around 32 weeks in a first pregnancy, and 35 weeks in subsequent pregnancies. In most cases this will be head down (cephalic). Babies can and do shift their position after this time, but it becomes increasingly less likely as they grow and have less room in which to move. There are some positions that a baby can adopt that necessitate delivery by Caesarean section if the position is maintained when you go into labour. These include transverse lie, when the baby lies across the abdomen, and shoulder presentation, when the baby's shoulder is the presenting part. Others such as unstable lie, when the baby keeps shifting its position at the end of pregnancy, and breech do not necessarily require an operative delivery, although this is a matter of opinion. Some consultants consider breech position to be an invariable indication for Caesarean section. Most others would consider it to be a high-risk situation that definitely requires delivery in a consultant unit with all the facilities for emergency section to hand. However this is largely because the skill of delivering breech babies, which used to be essential knowledge passed on from midwife to midwife throughout the years, has been lost (see Allison's account on page 6).

It is certainly true that a breech birth is potentially more dangerous than a cephalic one because of the pressure that the head may be subject to as it travels rapidly through the pelvis following the delivery of the baby's body. Further complications can be caused by the position of the baby's legs within the uterus. Breech delivery is traditionally done by a doctor, although midwives are trained in the theory of the various manoeuvres. It is therefore unusual these days for breech deliveries to be done at home. However it remains your right to have your baby at home whatever its presentation. The different types of provision that can be made are illustrated by Deborah's and Annie's stories of having their breech babies at home (see pages 125 and 127). Rosemary's account (page 123) of a quick and unexpected breech birth at home shows that it is not necessarily complicated.

You might contemplate having a breech baby at home if you cannot find a consultant prepared to allow you to try to have the baby vaginally or if your booked home birth baby remains persistently breech. If you do decide to have your breech baby at home you will want to be certain that your attendants are familiar with breech birth and that there are adequate plans for transfer to hospital if it should be necessary.

How you can help yourself

The best way to avoid these complications is to make sure that the baby changes position well before delivery, and there are several ways of doing this.

You may be able to tell if your baby is breech if you can feel a hard head bruising your ribs or if you get sudden sensations of urgency when the baby kicks you in the bladder. If the baby seems to be fixed in this position at around 32 weeks if it is your first baby, or 35 weeks if you have already had a child, you can take the following steps to help yourself. You can try and persuade the heaviest part of the baby – the head – to shift downwards by inverting yourself and allowing more room for a change in position. The best way of doing this is by holding yourself upside down in a swimming pool as often and for as long as is possible. You can also try the same sort of thing at home by lying with your hips higher than your head. This can either be on your back with a pile of cushions under your bottom and the soles of your feet on the floor, or by kneeling on the floor with your bottom in the air and your head resting on your arms on the floor. Try to sleep with three or four pillows under your bottom.

It can help to relax completely and talk to the baby, explaining why you want it to move. Visualise its head downwards. If the baby's bottom has engaged you will need to make the angle of inclination steeper in order to disengage it. You will probably know when the baby turns because it can feel like a big upheaval within your abdomen, which may even be painful.

If these techniques fail it is worth trying acupuncture or homeopathy. A homeopathic remedy is to take Pulsatilla 200 in two doses, two days apart in the 35th week. Consult a homeopath personally if this does not work. Acupuncture is particularly successful in turning babies. Consult an acupuncturist if the baby is breech at 35 weeks (or see my book *Alternative Maternity* for ways of using their technique at home).

If you should go into labour with a baby known to be breech and do not have assistance, stay upright or lean forward kneeling or adopt an all-fours position for the birth and allow the baby to deliver itself, which it can do. No one should touch the baby, until its head is born.

TWINS

Twin birth is possible at home but is not recommended because of the risk of the second twin turning into an unfavourable position once the first twin is delivered (although twin birth used to be customary at home). Even an independent midwife may not want to book you for a home birth with twins.

ANAEMIA

Anaemia is a result of a reduction in the quantity and quality of your haemoglobin (Hb) – the oxygen-carrying chemical in the red blood cells in your body. It is more likely to occur in the last three months of pregnancy when the baby's need for iron (a vital component of haemoglobin) is greatest. Suffering from anaemia can make you feel unusually tired.

Your blood is tested for its Hb level at several points in pregnancy and you will be considered anaemic if your level is below 11 g per 100 ml. The scale ranges from 14.7 g downwards; average Hb in non-pregnant women is 12.6 g. There will be serious concern if your Hb level drops to 9 g or lower. If you have anaemia at this level which is not improved by iron and folic acid supplementation, you will be under pressure to deliver in hospital. This is because low levels of iron can interfere with your blood clotting mechanism and might mean that you would have insufficient energy for labour and would make you prone to infection. Premature labour is more likely when a mother has anaemia. It also means that blood loss at delivery is potentially more hazardous as you cannot afford to lose much blood. However, the NICE draft guidelines for intrapartum care (p.162, June 2006) suggest that birth is recommended to take place in a consultant-led unit only if haemoglobin is under 8.5g/dl at the onset of labour.

How you can help yourself

If your haemoglobin level is seriously lowered you will be offered iron and folic acid supplements, either in tablet form or possibly by injection or intravenous infusion. The disadvantage of tablets is that they can make you feel sick or constipated, and they sometimes cause piles. This can make women reluctant to take them. Moreover the body does not absorb iron very well when it is given as a supplement, which is why it is often excreted in the form of jet-black stools. It is absorbed far more successfully from iron-rich foods in the diet, and it is a good idea to make a deliberate effort to include them in your diet in pregnancy. Foods that are rich in iron include lean red meat, especially kidney, watercress, wheat germ, dried fruit, dark green vegetables, cream, cottage cheese, cocoa, butterbeans and kidney beans.

If you are definitely anaemic or feel that you might be, you can take a herbal preparation called Floradix. It is available from healthfood shops in liquid and tablet form, and is extremely rich in natural iron. As iron is assimilated best in conjunction with vitamin C, you might like to try taking it with 1-4 g of vitamin C daily. Take double the stated dose of Floradix if your Hb is very low. You can get a cheaper form of iron combined with folic acid from the chemist. Fefol spansules are capsules filled with tiny slow-release pellets. Women often find them easier to tolerate than iron tablets. Iron absorption can be hindered by the consumption of bran, tea and coffee, so it is better to avoid these things. Drinking tea with meals is especially to be avoided. NDS Iron Plus, a low dose of iron that is well absorbed because it comes from food sources, may be the easiest to obtain (**www.ndshealthcare.com**).

Treatment from a herbalist, acupuncturist or homeopath can be very successful in eliminating anaemia.

PLACENTAL INSUFFICIENCY

Placental insufficiency is a condition where there is a reduction in the placenta's ability to sustain the baby. The placenta or afterbirth is the organ within the uterus where the baby's blood vessels exchange waste products from the baby's system for oxygen and other nutrients supplied by the mother's blood. If the placenta either does not develop normally or starts to deteriorate for some reason, the baby will go short of essential materials for growth. This will be apparent if your uterus is not growing at the expected rate and may be demonstrated by ultrasound (although see page 29 for relative degree of accuracy, and page 111 for concerns about ultrasound and inter uterine growth retardation). Placental insufficiency can be caused by raised blood pressure (see page 100), smoking, syphilis, diabetes and bleeding in pregnancy.

You can be reasonably sure that your placenta is functioning well if you are aware of the baby kicking frequently. You can check this for yourself by making your own kick chart. This can be done by charting the baby's movements, starting at the same time each day, e.g. 9 am. Count each separate movement you feel until you reach ten. Then make a note of the time. More than ten movements during 12 hours is a healthy sign. If the baby does not seem to move this often, or if the time by which it reaches ten each day is getting later and later every day, contact your midwife to get the baby monitored. However a recent study suggests that in fact kick charts are not especially good at predicting problems. Always trust your instinct; if you feel something is wrong, say so, even if you think that admitting to it may jeopardise your chances of a home birth.

Monitoring for placental insufficiency is usually by means of the cardiotocograph or belt monitor. This involves you lying down for half an hour while two belts with transducers are fastened around your abdomen. The baby's heartbeat is picked up by ultrasound and relayed to a machine which gives a printout. The other transducer measures the strength of any uterine contractions. The printout will supply information about the rate at which the fetal heart is beating and whether there is a good beat-to-beat variation. This should be enough to reassure everyone that your baby is well. If it does not, there are further tests that can be done to assess how well the placenta is functioning. There is also ultrasound; this cannot normally give you a good image of the placenta, although it can be done in specialist centres. If there is some doubt about how well the baby is growing you may be offered a scan at regular intervals in order to chart its progress, although see page 29 with regard to the accuracy of this form of monitoring.

How you can help yourself

If you are worried because you haven't felt the baby move for several hours, try taking three very deep breaths. The extra boost of oxygen often starts the baby moving. Failing this, try resting, relaxing as much as possible and lying on your left side. In this way the baby gets the best supply of blood to the placenta, and it will nearly always stimulate movement. Sometimes drinking a glass of very cold water can make the baby move. Get help if you are worried, although babies do often have periods of not moving for quite a long time, often at the 20-24 weeks stage.

If there is any question of the baby growing inadequately you should rest on your left for as long as possible each day. It may mean re-organising your life so that your reserves of energy are spread more evenly between you and the baby. It sometimes seems that when you are using a lot of energy the baby gets less oxygen. You may notice this if you don't feel the baby move much until you are sitting down or lying in bed. It also becomes especially important to eat well (see page 114), because a baby that is growing slowly may not be receiving the optimum amount of nutrients. It might help to take proprietary invalid foods like Complan if you really find it impossible to eat properly (further advice for those suffering with pregnancy sickness can be found in my book *Morning Sickness*). Increasing evidence is demonstrating the importance of a good diet in pregnancy.

Placental insufficiency can also be caused by maternal anxiety. This is particularly relevant to women who are anxious about whether they will be able to have their babies at home. It is difficult to relax under these conditions, but it is better for the baby if you try. It will help if you can avoid all those who are worried by home birth and speak to those who are in favour of the idea. Decide that you will only worry at a certain time of day and practise relaxation techniques regularly. Yoga classes could be especially helpful. You may be able to reassure yourself about your baby's growth by measuring your abdomen, no more often than weekly. If it really seems that your baby is not growing well bearing in mind that babies normally vary in birth weight between 5 and 10 pounds – contact a nutritionist or acupuncturist for specialist help.

IF YOU ARE OVERDUE

You may be able to avoid this becoming a problem by bringing the date of the first day of your last monthly period forward, so that your estimated date of delivery is thought to be a week later than it really is (as described in the story on page 20). Clearly you can only do this before you start receiving your antenatal care.

Research has shown that babies can safely go to 44 weeks of pregnancy if their condition is monitored every few days.[32] The NICE draft guidelines state that women who decline induction should be offered increased antenatal monitoring consisting of a twice-weekly CTG and ultrasound estimation of maximum amniotic pool depth[33]. However you may be under pressure to go into hospital for induction if the baby is 10 days or so late, depending on local policy. There is no way that you can be forced into hospital, and you should just refuse politely if you do not want labour started artificially. However, if you are more than 10 days late, you may be feeling keen to get on with labour yourself. The following suggestions are ways to start things off, although you may prefer not to use them, feeling that a baby will come when it is ready and that labour will be smoother for waiting. Your midwife may offer to sweep your membranes, this is where she puts a gloved finger into your cervix and sweeps it around the top so that the lower membranes become detached. Two studies suggest that sweeping the membranes is an effective method of induction of labour in women who are overdue as it puts two thirds of them into labour within three days.[34] Bear in mind though, that the average (uninterrupted) length of pregnancy is 41 weeks 2 days. Read more about sweeping membranes on the Association of Radical Midwives (ARM) website at **www.midwifery.org.uk**.

How you can help yourself

Frequent sex may initiate labour at full-term by means of the prostaglandins in semen. You should remain on your back for half an hour afterwards. You can also try a purgative such as a hot curry, or a third of a tumbler of castor oil mixed with orange juice. These can tip you into labour, as can an enema, but you may be left feeling weak as a result.

A homeopathic remedy for starting labour is to take Caulophyllum 30 every half hour until contractions are well-established. If contractions slow down once you stop taking it, you should continue to take it throughout labour. Otherwise you could visit an acupuncturist, herbalist or reflexologist, all of whom may be able to start labour off gently, although you may need several appointments.

Ruptured membranes

If your waters have gone, you know the baby's head is engaged and the liquor is clear and the baby does not seem to be in any distress, you can just wait for contractions to begin or try any one of the methods of inducing labour that do not involve direct contact with the vagina (see above).

If you report it to your midwife and contractions do not start within 24 hours you may be under pressure to go in for induction because many consultants believe that you or the baby are at risk of infection. However, the NICE guidelines state that women with premature rupture of membranes should be offered expectant management for up to 96 hours before offering to induce labour, because 86 per cent of women will go into spontaneous labour within 24 hours. Thereafter 91 per cent will have started labour within 47 hours, and 94 per cent by the time membranes have been ruptured for 95 hours, leaving 6 per cent not yet in labour. Evidence that awaiting events at home is safe can be found in *Home Management for Mothers with PROM at Term is Safe*[35]. Linda's story on page 176 gives an account of her experience of waiting for labour to begin following ruptured membranes, with an interesting comment that shows how old knowledge has been rediscovered.[36]

You can reduce the risk of infection by taking 8 garlic perles and 1 gramme of vitamin C, several times a day and being scrupulous about hygiene. Nothing should be placed in the vagina, you should shower rather than have a bath and take your temperature every four hours. Drink plenty to replace the fluid you are losing. If you develop a fever, or the fluid you are losing smells unpleasant or becomes coloured you should get medical help immediately.

WOMEN'S STORIES

"I nearly missed Guy's birth myself, it was so quick. I awoke feeling very bright at 5.50 am one morning and decided to make a cup of tea. When I reached the kettle I had a very

strange pain – not a contraction but very low down. It lasted just a couple of seconds, then happened again a few minutes later. I thought it was just the beginning of labour and decided to wake my husband. We had to get organised early so as to get my in-laws to come and look after the older children while we went to hospital.

"Dale greeted my news as he would anything at 6 am. But as I sat on the bed prodding him the pains became very severe and I couldn't apply my breathing techniques so got a bit distraught. We rushed downstairs and rang the parents, then decided I couldn't wait for them and I'd better go in an ambulance. Then I realised I couldn't wait for that either and we'd have to go by car, with the children. Dale ran upstairs and hauled them out of bed, only to be called down again urgently as I felt the baby descending rapidly. He carried me upstairs, plonked me on the bed and ran down to call the midwife, doctor, anyone.

"Meanwhile, with one dazed, little pyjama-clad boy holding each of my hands, I lay on my side and chatted calmly whilst breathing slowly and deeply allowing the baby to slide gently out. Owen (five and a half years old) said 'Look Mummy, there's the baby's feet' (I won't write down what I thought). There had been no indication of a breech presentation, but I checked and, sure enough, there were two feet, and further up . . . 'What's this Owen?' – 'It's a willy, Mummy!'

"Dale arrived back in the bedroom to see that the body was born as far as the shoulders but what should we do next? He questioned the cleanliness of his hands and checked around the neck for the cord and position of the chin. Then with no effort at all on my part, the head slipped out, wearing the placenta like a floppy hat! The time was 6.20 am – only half an hour since I'd woken up!

"The ambulance men, midwife and doctor then arrived in quick succession. We were declared fit and healthy. Guy was fed and cuddled, then they all went away and that was that.

"It was a jolly exciting morning and I realised many of the benefits of a home delivery. What I did miss was the big production drama of the trip to the hospital, the timing of contractions, the mounting excitement and 'Push – push harder – push', etc. But how nice to have hardly felt any pain and not be tired out. It was a lovely family occasion too. Owen had plenty to talk about at school that week, and little Hugh still asks about the funny man who came into our bedroom.

"I would like to know, why I had no contractions though (the pains were obviously the cervix dilating), and was it just that I'd had several babies or is there another reason for precipitate labours? Whatever the reason it was an amazing experience."

Rosemary

"My baby boy was born at home after six hours of labour. He was a foot presentation. I had no drugs, no episiotomy, no interference. There were no problems. I was relaxed and happy. Two midwives helped to deliver him, a doctor was in the other room but was not needed. This was my first baby, and we are both doing well. He is happy and contented – sleeps through the night with me in bed, and is breastfed of course!"

Deborah Wilson

"Our problem was that our baby was breech presentation whenever I was examined by my doctor or midwife, but did move quite freely at other times. Having only been with my doctor for a few months, neither she nor my midwife had much confidence in me, and vice versa. My midwife, Mrs O., did not like home deliveries, although she did say she had participated in some.

"Our local hospital's policy is that any breech presentation at 35 weeks must be notified to a consultant, for Caesarean section at 37 weeks if the baby has not turned. No manual turning is ever attempted. I wanted to wait until I was in labour before deciding whether to try for a breech delivery or not, or to see if the baby would turn at the last minute, as my previous baby had done. (Unfortunately she turned the wrong way whilst I was in labour and I had an emergency breech delivery without anaesthetic but an episiotomy and forceps.) I was offered a forceps delivery by the hospital a day after the baby was due, but I was reluctant to agree as by this time my husband and I had decided to try for a 'normal' breech delivery. We found we couldn't get any information about this. Nobody we spoke to could help and we were advised that the hospital knew best. We were told that the consultants would let us deliver only if I refused a Caesarean section, but only with forceps and not by my midwife. I had to go into the consultant unit and not into the GP unit, which we would have preferred. I felt unable to agree to this and I refused and stated my determination for a home delivery, much to Mrs O.'s horror. All I knew was that breech deliveries were better done by squatting, but that was the only information given. I was scared stiff about delivering a baby virtually without medical aid, just with Mrs O. who said that she wouldn't leave us although she didn't agree with the idea.

"On December 14 I went into labour and called Mrs O. She came with another midwife. You should have seen the look on her face when she examined me to find I was three-quarters of the way there and the baby was head presentation. We were pretty sure the baby would turn if given enough time. Mrs O. delivered Maria, our baby girl, at 5.19 that evening, and from what she said we gathered that she had only ever helped deliver one baby at home, and that when she was a student midwife. I hope we have helped change her mind about home birth, as we feel that more women should be given the choice, not only of place of birth but way too. I would have gone to hospital if I could be assured of delivering without interference, but the hospital 'washed their hands of us'. We had to play the game their way or not at all."

Jackie Murphy

"When I became pregnant for the second time I was determined to have as good an experience as I'd had the first time round when my daughter Lucy, despite being in a breech position, had been delivered by Yehudi Gordon in a wonderfully calm, magical atmosphere – without forceps etc. – in a hospital. I wanted this baby to be born at home and, perhaps with the thought that it too might be breech, I booked with Caroline Flint, an independent midwife. As the months went by it became clear that no. 2 was also going to be a breech baby but having been through it before, I had complete confidence in my own and Caroline's ability and was clear I wanted to stay at home. Caroline also arranged for another midwife, experienced in breech deliveries, and a GP to be present which, with her partner Lorna, probably meant that I was better attended than in most hospitals.

"My labour started with my waters breaking spontaneously at 7.30. Caroline arrived at 8.30 as my contractions were starting. It was a perfect labour – contractions built up in strength gradually through the morning as I carried on as normal, and at 1.30 I moved upstairs as the hard work was really beginning. Two and a half hours later and, in a standing position, supported by Peter, my beautiful Katie was born – all 8 lb 11 oz of her – bottom first and no more than a small tear to show for it. The experience was everything we had hoped for, different from Lucy's birth but with just the same magic.

"I've now had two breech deliveries, one in hospital and one at home, but both the way I wanted them, without unnecessary intervention and with the love and support of everyone around me. It can be done!"

Annie Francis, *AIMS Journal* (Annie has since had another daughter at home, head first this time.)

9   the birth

Guidelines about labouring at home are not really necessary, as the beauty of the situation is that you are free to do what you want, as and when you want. As one woman said with glee, **"I was in control, no one at all could make me do anything I didn't want to."**

You will probably have already discussed with the midwife at what stage she would like to be called. This is obviously up to you and the way you are feeling at the time. Depending on the circumstances you may find it reassuring to have her come and check your progress and then perhaps go again, leaving some way of contacting her. Some midwives arrange to return at a certain time, provided they have not been called before.

There are few instances where you should call your midwife or doctor immediately:

- If you are in labour before 36 weeks. A baby below this gestational age may have difficulty breathing, may be unable to suck and loses heat very easily, no matter how well dressed.
- If your waters go with a gush and you know the baby's head to be high or not fixed in the pelvis. This is because there is a very slight risk that the cord may prolapse (descend before the head) and become compressed against the bony pelvis by the head, thus cutting off the supply of oxygen to the baby. This only happens in 1 in 400 cases, and the most often in premature or induced labour. In this situation call your midwife or doctor immediately and lie down in the knee-chest position, with your head on your crossed arms and your bottom as high as possible in the air. This takes the pressure off the cervix so that, if the cord has prolapsed, it will not be pinched. Once it has been checked you can carry on as normal.
- If your waters go and the fluid is coloured or contains lumps, particularly if it is greeny-black, as this can be an indication of

current fetal distress.

Lightly meconium stained liquor alone does not indicate a requirement for continuous electronic fetal monitoring or transfer to a consultant unit from midwifery-led unit or home.

- If you are bleeding and the amount is sufficient to soak a sanitary pad.

GETTING THINGS READY

You might like to take some of the following steps. None are essential, apart from making sure that you have the room temperature up to 25 degrees Centigrade by the time the baby is born.

- Get the pvc-backed fabric, sheets and towels into the room in which you think you will give birth, although you may change your mind about this.
- Make sure the baby clothes and nappy are ready.
- Make up the crib and put a hot water bottle in it.
- Bring in extra cushions, pillows, bean bags or birth ball.
- Make sure you have something to lean over – an ironing board with a pillow on it can be useful.
- Make lots of tea/raspberry leaf tea.
- Drink and eat easily digested food freely. Don't worry if you are sick; it is quite normal in labour.
- Have a bucket or two lined with a bin-liner in case they are needed, for vomiting or as a potty.
- If labour is going slowly, you might want to spend some time preparing something to eat or baking a cake for when it is over.
- Put newspaper down if walking around with leaking membranes, or use a child-size disposable nappy.
- Make sure that you have film or batteries and memory in your camera.
- If using TENS, have a bath or shower and then put it on while still in early labour.
- An open fire is nice, if applicable.
- Pin up your birth plan if you have one.
- Make an inviting space for the midwives.

Try to conserve your energy as far as possible. It can be a good idea just to carry on as normal, as many of the women in the case histories did. Try and ignore the contractions until you are forced to stop and take notice of them. If you start labour in the middle of the night, you should try and get some sleep if at all possible. You might find that taking a couple of paracetamol and a hot drink helps. This will not slow labour if it really is underway, but can get you over false starts without exhausting you unnecessarily.

When your contractions need attention you may be helped by the application of a hot water bottle, frequent changes of position, a bath, rocking yourself to and fro or rotating your hips in a circle, and massage from your partner or a friend. You might want to put some essential oil such as lavender or clary sage in the massage oil or in the bath water (more information about coping with labour is available in my book *Labour Pain*).

LABOUR ITSELF

If you have not already called the midwife before, you might want to give her a ring when contractions are every three minutes or so. This is really your decision and will depend on your circumstances, the speed with which she can reach you, and your relationship with her. The baby is more likely to arrive quickly if it is not your first. Always ring if you are frightened or feel that you cannot cope or if you feel that something is wrong.

If contractions slow or stop when your midwife arrives, ask her to check you and come back later. Many midwives are happy to stay in another room and let you get on with labour, checking you and the baby from time to time and being on hand if needed. If your midwife is not prepared to do this and you feel that her feelings about home birth are having a deleterious effect on your labour, ring the supervisor or the answering service and ask for a different midwife. She will probably be happier not to be there, and your labour is more important than possibly hurting her feelings. Obviously, though, it is better to get this sorted out before labour starts (see page 158) and on some occasions it may not be possible to have a change of midwife. It is best to have sympathetic people with you if at all possible.

Make as much noise as you want. Groaning, shouting and swearing can all really help the baby out – although your partner should be warned that it may sound quite alarming. Grunting is normal in the second stage. Curiously, children do not seem to be woken by these noises, often appearing uncannily after the baby has been born.

Once you are in the second stage you will need to prepare the actual birthing area. The second stage may be signalled in various ways — an uncontrollable urge to push, grunting at the height of a contraction, feeling of a large, round object in the rectum, fresh bleeding, or involuntary opening of the bowels. Any of these should mean that someone should put down the plastic, covered by sheets or towels, on the bed or floor. Your midwife may bring incontinence pads with her, but they are not necessarily large enough to soak up all the blood, mucus and amniotic fluid that is inevitably delivered with the baby. (Bedclothes, carpets, etc., that are soiled can be cleaned up by careful cleaning and rinsing with a biological detergent, oxygen bleach or hydrogen peroxide.)

Your position should be dictated by what you find most help-ful. This may be on all fours, squatting supported by furniture or your companions, hanging round the neck of your partner, stand-ing, kneeling upright or even on your side. It is better to avoid posi-tions where you are resting on your bottom or back as you have to push against gravity and your coccyx is not free to move back out of the way of the baby's head.

Once born, the baby should be wrapped in a warm towel. Then, after the placenta is delivered, you can if you want, both have a bath together. After that you can get into bed and celebrate, and let everyone else clear up around you.

EQUIPMENT

There is very little equipment that is absolutely essential for giv-ing birth, as those women who have delivered unexpectedly have discovered. Probably the most important thing is some form of heating or, failing that, warm wrappings to prevent the baby becoming cold after the birth. A newborn baby can lose body heat very rapidly, especially if it is still wet. However there are things which may be useful in making a planned home birth more com-fortable and less messy, although mess is not the overwhelming problem it is sometimes made out to be.

Once you are booked for a home birth your midwife will give

you a list of things that she would like you to provide. You might also like to collect some other things that other women have found helpful when they had their babies at home.

For the bed

- Clean sheets.
- Large plastic sheeting from ironmongers or garden centre or you can buy waterproof mattress covers. These can be less slippery than polythene. You could also use the disposable bed mats sold for bed-wetting children.
- Biological washing powder for washing sheets or cleaning stained carpets. The oxygen-based bleaches and hydrogen peroxide can be very useful.

For you

- Large T-shirt or man's shirt for labour. Clean nighties.
- Maternity-size sanitary pads. Nursing bras.
- Old pants or sanitary knickers to keep pads in place (both bras and knickers available from NCT Maternity Sales).
- Child-size waterproof-backed disposable nappies if waters leak in labour.
- Large portable mirror to watch birth.
- Perfume (although very strong perfumes and soaps can put the baby off feeding).
- Preprepared meals such as soup or anything you think you might like to eat or drink in labour or afterwards.
- Ice cubes – plain and made from fruit-juice or raspberry-leaf tea.
- Fructose tablets or powder (this is more slowly absorbed than glucose).
- Isotonic sports drinks – but avoid those containing aspartame.
- Flexible straws.
- Bath essence.
- Hair ties.
- Towel.
- Hot water bottle.
- Warm socks.
- Two clean flannels.

- Talcum powder.
- Rescue remedy.
- Water spray.

For the baby

- Baby clothes – nightie or babygro, vest, newborn size disposable nappies or muslin or terry nappies, cardigan, hat, bootees, mittens, shawl or wrap. Put clothes on radiator to warm at the start of labour.
- Crib – made up.
- Clean towels.
- Hot-water bottle to warm crib.
- Baby lotion or plain soap.
- Pleated cotton wool.

For the midwife

- Birth plan if necessary.
- Clean towel and soap.
- Nail brush.
- Handbowl.
- Thermometer.
- Two buckets lined with bin liners (useful for rubbish, but also for being sick into or as a potty if necessary).
- Plastic bin-liners.
- Cupboard top or small table to lay out equipment.
- Angle-poise lamp or torch.

Other equipment

- Bean bag.
- Birth ball.
- Plenty of pillows and cushions.
- Music.
- Light reading, video or other entertainment for early hours of morning.
- Candles.
- Flowers.
- Newspaper (said to be for the midwife to read but can be

useful for covering carpets).
- Old towels or sheets for the same purpose.
- Hot water for copious cups of tea (you may need to get in extra milk).
- Exciting snacks for midwives.
- Phone numbers of your midwife, doctor, person to take care of children (overnight bag for children including teddy), labour supporter, paramedics, etc., by phone.
- Any herbal or homeopathic remedies wanted (see below).
- Paracetamol tablets.
- Celebratory drink.
- Transcutaneous nerve stimulator (TENS).
- Aromatherapy and massage oils. Almond oil is good for massage and as a base for the essential oils.
- Essential oil burner if desired.
- Birthing tub.
- Rope suspended from ceiling (for hanging on to in second stage).
- Notebook and pen.
- Water spray.
- Clock.
- Food for attendants.
- Camera loaded with film or digital camera; fast film for if the baby is born at night and you do not want to use a flash.
- Disinfectant (a floral one can make things smell less clinical).
- Kitchen paper.
- Tissues.
- Plasticine or Blu-tac to plug the bath overflow to make it deeper.
- Muslin with which to make compresses.
- Essential items in a bag in case of transfer.

Alternative remedies

Homeopathic remedies are available from healthfood shops and some chemists in 6C potency; other potencies are available from homeopathic pharmacies. You can also order other potencies from Galens (see Useful Addresses) who supply large tablets which dissolve quickly, useful in labour. Suggested remedies include Arnica 200, Pulsatilla 6, Caullophyllum 30, Kali Phos, Gelsemium,

Phosphorus, while Mag Phos is useful for afterpains.

Herbal remedies are available by post from Baldwin's. Their use is described in my book *Alternative Maternity*:

- Goldenseal tincture or dried herb.
- Calendula or hypercal tincture for helping to heal stitches.
- Arnica cream for bruised perineum.
- Garlic perles to be taken in combination with vitamin C to combat infection.
- Slippery elm powder to make soothing poultices for sore nipples or stitches.
- Vitamin E or comfrey oil to bind the slippery elm powder with.
- Raspberry leaf tea and tablets.
- Cayenne pepper, ground ivy tincture, black cohosh tincture and blue cohosh tincture in case of haemorrhage.
- Bach flower rescue remedy.

Equipment carried by the midwife

It can be a good idea to check that the midwife is carrying the following items, which you may need in labour, although this should be done tactfully.

- Oxygen.
- Ambubag/intubation equipment.
- Urinary catheter.
- Entonox and pethidine. Ask how much Entonox they carry – small cylinders do not last long.
- Ergometrine/Syntometrine for injection.
- Pethidine/Narcan (you may be required to get your own prescription for this if you feel you might need it – Narcan is to counteract the sedative effects of pethidine on the baby.
- Materials for suturing.
- Doppler/Sonicaid – this is a portable ultrasonic monitor carried by some midwives and useful for listening to the baby's heart when you are in the bath or in alternative positions. If she does not own or carry one she may be able to get one from the labour ward when you are in labour.
- Intravenous fluid set.

- Bed pan.
- Cord scissors, clamp and ligature.
- Local anaesthetic.
- Scales.
- Warming pad.
- Episiotomy scissors.

Find out how many people will attend the labour; ideally there should be two.

Obstetric emergency provision

The obstetric flying squads have been disbanded and replaced by paramedics. It is sensible to find out what provision is made for an obstetric emergency – how soon an ambulance could reach you, how long it would take to get you to hospital, and what experience the paramedics have of birth. Ask what equipment they carry to assist mothers and babies in difficulties, including neonatal resuscitation equipment and portable incubator. Find out from your midwives what experience they have had in dealing with obstetric or paediatric emergencies at home and how the service provision worked on those occasions.

WATER BIRTH

Water birth is considered here because, although it is obtainable in many hospitals and, with negotiation, may be available in more, the one place you can be certain of having your baby in water is at home. The advantages are that it can be very relaxing, the water can afford some degree of pain relief, your perineal skin becomes softer and more supple, reducing the chance of an episiotomy, and the babies seem to enjoy it. On the other hand, if you hire a tub it involves prior organisation and expense and your midwives may not be experienced in helping women to give birth in water.

Some suggestions from those who have been involved in home water births include:

- Make enquiries early in pregnancy. Investigate as many designs of tubs as possible and try them out if you can. Consider whether you might be better off installing a new large or oval bath in your bathroom, which one midwife, experienced in water birth, feels would be just as good and has the advantage of being permanent. This would minimise the problems of floor strength, water heating and disposal. You can plug the overflow with plasticine or Blu-tac to make it deeper.

- Discuss the question of water birth with your midwives or doctor. If they will not consider it, you might want to think about employing an independent midwife.
- Check arrangements for filling the tub and for heating the water. Some tubs have thermostatically controlled water heaters which will keep the water at a constant 39 degrees Centigrade. Some have covers which will keep the water warm while not in use. Others just need topping up with very hot water; because the body of water is large and the room temperature quite high, this is adequate to maintain the temperature.
- If your bedroom floor will not take the weight of the filled tub, it has to stay downstairs.
- Have the wiring checked by an electrician or electricity board – you need to be careful when combining water and electricity. You should have trip-fuses installed.
- Have a dress rehearsal. You might find that you need a friend there as well as your partner.
- Make sure that you have an alternative dry space for labour. You cannot be sure that you will want to be in water when you are in labour and you may need to get out suddenly if there is any sign of fetal distress. A Sonicaid is useful for checking the fetal heart while you remain in the tub.
- Ensure there is adequate ventilation in the room, which can get very hot. Occasionally babies need to be taken into a cooler atmosphere to start breathing. If the room is not hot, it needs to be up to at least 25 degrees Centigrade for the birth.
- Some midwives have a policy of not allowing a woman into the pool before she is 5 cm dilated, because there is evidence that this can slow labour. It does not seem logical that women can be encouraged to get in a bath but not a pool at this stage. Moreover a three year study of water births in Birmingham by Lyn Brown[37] states that although it may slow or stop labour, it is not a reason to restrict a woman from the

pool. If it does slow or stop, she can leave the pool and re-enter when it starts again.

- You may enjoy essential oils such as lavender or clary sage in the water.
- Once the baby is born, trust to your instinct about when to bring it into the air. However, if the cord stops pulsating the baby should be lifted out immediately. Once out of the water the baby should be dried thoroughly and kept warm (he or she can be kept warm initially in warm, wet blankets). You may want to have him or her back in once the third stage is over.

Some of the anxieties felt by people who have not witnessed water births centre around the health of the baby; they fear that it might drown, or that it might be infected by faecal matter from the mother contaminating the water. There is also concern that water might get into the uterus if the third stage takes place in water.

Midwives who have attended water births are certain that it is physiologically safe and impossible for a baby to drown before it has taken a breath in air. Tests by microbiologists at Maidstone hospital show that it is safe as far as infection is concerned. The staff there believe in administering an enema or suppositories before the birth, although others consider that it is inevitable and even desirable that a baby is colonised by his mother's germs as soon as possible. There is no evidence to show that anyone has suffered from water entering the uterus, but it may be a good idea to remain upright until the placenta is delivered if you are staying in water for the third stage. Be prepared for the water to turn red suddenly as the placenta is delivered. Some midwives prefer the third stage out of water in order to assess blood loss.

"My water birth really came about as a practical measure because I have a downstairs bathroom and my midwife was not keen on my going downstairs for a bath after the delivery. I discussed giving birth under water with her while I was pregnant and she attended a seminar on the subject, so she was quite happy.

"When I went into labour I didn't get into the water straight away but carried on as normal, cooking supper for the boys and James, putting the children to bed and straightening things out. I really enjoyed that.

"When my waters broke and the contractions got strong, I

got into the bath. I would like to stress that I am not especially small at 5 feet 9 inches tall, and I was quite large. Our bath is of average size but I didn't feel cramped or stuck at all. I stayed there rocking from side to side which was really comforting in itself. I just watched the water swirling over my abdomen and relaxed. I didn't feel any of the burning and tension in my stomach that I had felt with the other two in hospital. It was a completely different dimension, and the labour had a different feel to it.

"I was completely in tune with what was happening, and when I felt the baby's head coming down I told the midwife and she suggested I gave a push. I knew exactly the right time to do it, gave a push and his head was born. Very little effort was needed, then he was born, as easily and as quickly as that. He stayed under water for a short while and the midwife kept a finger on his cord to ensure that it was still pulsating. Then I lifted him on to my stomach. He was all pink and gorgeous and he popped his eyes open. He had his first feed in the bath very shortly after he was born.

"I can't remember much about the third stage but everything happened in the bath. All the midwife had to do was take the placenta out of the bath and all the rest of the mess flowed down the drain. She just re-ran the bath and we got in again and were extremely comfortable.

"After he was born my two little boys woke up and came in – they thought it was great that his birthplace was our bath. He was nearly 8 pounds, the same as the others had been but, unlike with them, I had no episiotomy and no stitches, just a tiny tear which mended itself. Ever since his birth Benedict has loved water; when we went on holiday to Spain when he was 11 months old he spent most of the time standing up to his shoulders in the Mediterranean. I don't know if it is coincidence but he always loved being bathed as a baby, whereas the others hated it.

"I would really recommend it, but you can't make people do things – they've really got to want to do them themselves."

Lesley Redmond

CHILDREN PRESENT

Giving birth at home provides the opportunity for your children to be present at the birth if you wish. Both you and they may have strong feelings about this, although clearly you should not have them there if you do not want them to be. Their wishes about avoiding it should be respected too.

You may not want them there if you feel that you will be putting their feelings before yours, are likely to be concerned about the way they are reacting, if their presence is likely to make you more restrained or quieter than you otherwise would be, or if you do not want to risk them seeing you apparently distressed or out of control. Remember, it can be hard for them to watch someone they love in labour.

On the other hand, you may feel that it is something that they really should not miss, or they may themselves be very keen to be there, or you may feel that it would be the best possible start to their new relationship and that it may provide a good basis for their own childbearing in years to come. Discuss it with them well beforehand and make sure that the idea of flexibility is introduced. It is useful if they realise they may not be present, either because they may not be there at the time or because you may change your mind when you are actually in labour. There is also a chance that complications will make it impossible or undesirable.

It is hard to know what the long-term effects of seeing their brother's or sister's birth may have on a child. In the short term they seem to accept it happily and be glad about it. Probably the least desirable situation is for a child to be able to hear what is going on but not be able to see it. It may be important to make sure children are asleep while you are in labour; if not, you should see that they are either with you or with someone who can look after them and explain what is happening.

If you do intend to have your children with you at the birth, talk to your community midwives about it before you go into labour. Not all will be keen on the idea, but very few would actually send a child away once there. It is important to have some contingency arrangement in case things do not go according to plan. This might be someone who would come to your house and look after them in another room − but it would have to be someone who would not mind missing the birth itself. Otherwise you need someone who will take the children home with them, in the middle of the night if necessary.

It is very interesting to note that in most of the labour reports of mothers with existing children, the new babies are born at night when the other children are asleep. If they wake at all it is only once the baby has been born, even though there may have been quite a high level of noise and a lot of activity.

One experienced midwife thinks that you can almost rely on labour really getting under way after the children are asleep – further evidence of the powerful effect the subconscious can have on the process of labour (also demonstrated by the high proportion of women who start labour during the night after being admitted to hospital for induction the following morning).

Being present at, or immediately after, the birth does seem to help the other children accept the baby, but it does not guarantee that there will not be problems of jealousy.

"It was nice to be there. I didn't like it when she came out all white – I thought she would be pink. Daddy picked her up and then I held her and Daddy went down and got a drink, then I took her into my bedroom. I didn't mind Mummy making a noise. I felt very pleased because I was hoping she was a sister. I don't think William would have enjoyed it. I don't think he would have been interested. It was kind of special. When I went to school my friends were pleased and talked to me about it, and my teachers were glad."

Eleanor (aged seven)

"It meant a lot to me to have her there and to share something with her. I would not have minded if the boys had been there but I think it would have been chaos if they had all been there. Eleanor so much wanted a sister – it was really special for her."

Catherine Gash

"Eleanor was not necessarily going to be at the birth, but was awake while Catherine was in labour and stayed up to be there (Rosamund was born at 10.30 pm). She was frequently offered the opportunity to leave if she wanted. Catherine reassured her several times that she was all right, despite the noise she was making. Shortly after Rosamund's cord had been clamped,

Eleanor took her, wrapped in a towel, to show her bedroom to her. They were found in there with Rosamund tucked carefully under the duvet, listening to Eleanor telling her about her family and counting to her. Eleanor continued to look after her and explained everything to her, keeping up a running commentary which included their mother being stitched. My final memory is of seeing all three of them in bed together, relaxing after the great excitement."

Midwife

"When we discovered that I was expecting our third baby, Billy and I decided to opt for a home birth. The births of our daughters Stephanie and Frances in hospital had been uncomplicated and gentle, but we both firmly believed that the birth should be a family celebration in the home, not taking place in the clinical surroundings of a labour ward. I had been attended by the same experienced and very sympathetic midwife for both deliveries and she supported our decision.

"I considered myself very fortunate to be accepted for a home birth by the first GP I approached. All was proceeding well until I developed pleurisy which developed into pneumonia in the 18th week of pregnancy. I was hospitalised and subjected to X-rays and lung scans to exclude the possibility of a pulmonary embolism. I was very anxious despite assurances that they would not harm my unborn child. This experience strengthened my resolve to give birth naturally at home where I could be sure that neither myself nor my baby would be exposed to any unnecessary interference.

"Within a month I had made a full recovery, my baby was kicking strongly and had grown noticeably. The pregnancy progressed well without further complications and at dawn in the 39th week of my pregnancy, my waters broke. The sun had already risen, the birds were singing and Billy and I felt great excitement at the thought of seeing our new baby soon. When the girls woke I told them that their brother or sister would be born that day. (They were so convinced that it would be a girl that they had called it Eleanor throughout the pregnancy).

"I telephoned my midwife Christine, then we all had breakfast together. I packed my mother off for her driving lesson and Billy took Frances out to the shops. I felt very calm and wanted everyone to go about their business as normal until I needed their support. The baby was very active and I was experiencing mild contractions. At 10 am Christine arrived to examine me – I had been comfortably playing with Stephanie and was very surprised to discover that I was already 6 cm dilated.

"By now it was obvious that it was going to be another scorching hot day and I was very glad of the fan we had installed in the bedroom. We opened the windows and closed the curtains so the room was cool, dim and quiet. My contractions were becoming stronger and more frequent and I was glad of Billy's cool hands rubbing the base of my spine. Christine asked me whether we would like the girls to be present at the birth and we decided that they would appreciate being included. They had been involved throughout the pregnancy by listening to the heartbeat with Christine's Sonicaid, feeling the baby kick and accompanying me to antenatal appointments so it felt natural to include them.

"Stephanie was keen to help and kept me cool by washing my face and neck with a cool flannel. Frances' contribution was gentle hugs and kisses at regular intervals. Christine explained that I was having to work very hard and they did not appear too disturbed by my moans and groans. Their presence helped me enormously – their humorous comments reduced the tension and provided a distraction from the pain.

"Christine was monitoring the well-being of both myself and the baby throughout, encouraging me when I needed support, but giving Billy and me time alone together when I was coping. I remained mobile, leaning over the bed and or hanging around Billy's neck during contractions. As I neared the end of the first stage I began to feel very hot and bad tempered and decided to move to the shower to cool down. The girls were also getting impatient so they retired to the garden. Frances had just fallen asleep in her grandma's arms when I felt the urge to push and Christine called them up to the bathroom. I was using Entonox to help me to 'let go' and still using the shower between contractions. In my drunken haze I was aware of Billy in the bath beside me, and the girls standing quietly with Christine. The contractions became intense, I leant back against the tiles, bent my knees and pushed down hard. I heard Christine telling the girls that she could see the baby's ears

appearing and, with the next contraction, the baby was delivered. I reached down to take our daughter in my arms. I looked
around and saw that Billy was crying and Christine had tears in
her eyes. We hugged. Baby Eleanor lay quiet and pink in my
arms.

"Christine waited for the umbilical cord to stop pulsating and
then Billy cut the cord as he had at Stephanie and Frances'
births. Once the placenta was delivered we filled the bath so
that Eleanor and I could relax together and allow the girls to
admire their new sister. Billy then wrapped Eleanor in a warm
towel and she turned her head to face her sisters – three pairs
of wide eyes taking each other in. It was a very special moment
which will never be forgotten, one which convinced us that
their presence had been very important. Stephanie and Frances
then followed the midwives into the bedroom to watch Eleanor
being examined and weighed. We were all surprised to discover
that she was a bouncing 9 lb!

"The next few hours flashed by with visits from the midwives,
GP and family, and the girls buzzed around the cot eagerly
awaiting the next opportunity to hold Eleanor. Once we had
enjoyed a well-deserved meal and the girls had been tucked up
in bed, Billy and I sat together holding Eleanor, watching her
constantly changing expressions, admiring her perfect features.
Eleanor had fed well and was sleeping peacefully so we
returned to bed, tired but elated. It was the end of a long, hot
day, the sun was setting and we could hear the blackbird's
evening song – a perfect ending to a very special day."

Hilary Adam

10   do-it-yourself delivery

"My husband and I are curious as to what the authorities could do if we decided at the time not to call the midwife, as I would very much like my husband to deliver my baby and I know that the midwife would not be prepared to take a back seat if we called her. This is something we feel very strongly about and I feel safe and more comfortable having my husband there instead of the midwife – who, incidentally, is still trying to make me go into hospital."

It is difficult not to feel sympathy with the mother who wrote this. However, do-it-yourself delivery is not recommended because of the slight risk of either you or the baby needing the specialised skill or equipment of the midwife. Moreover you can be prosecuted if it can be proved that you intended to deliver a baby when not qualified as either a midwife or a doctor, although prosecution is intended for those fraudulently claiming to be qualified. A statement clarifying this was made in September 2002 by Jacqui Smith MP, the Minister of State at the Department of Health, when she wrote to Julia Drown MP as follows:

Attending a woman in childbirth, as opposed to general support given by partners and relatives, has been an offence against the protected function of midwifery since the Midwives Act 1902 and the fines [£5,000] are set at a level to reflect the seriousness of the offence. By 'attend' we mean, 'assume responsibility for care' and this is not intended to outlaw husbands, partners and relatives whose presence and support during childbirth are extremely important.

Some midwives suspect that their aid has been dispensed with deliberately when they arrive at the home of a newly-born baby too late, although if the parents are adamant that it arrived without warning there is nothing that the midwife can do. However it does mean that parents whose baby has arrived genuinely without warning are sometimes subject to interrogation, adding to their shock and bewilderment and making them feel very uneasy.

If you are booked for a home birth you will at least be expecting to have your baby at home. But babies can and do arrive before the midwife, so it is important to have some idea of what to do. This is not so much because such a baby will need help – a baby that is born that quickly is generally fine and so is its mother – but in order that you can feel calm about what is happening. Knowing what to do in this situation will not only give you confidence but it can also help you visualise the baby's progress in labour when the baby arrives more slowly, and means that you can cooperate with your midwife at the time of delivery.

You might realise that your baby was arriving suddenly if you had some contractions and felt an overwhelming desire to push, or felt the baby's head in the birth canal (a sensation something like a grapefruit in your rectum). Ring the midwife or doctor if you have not already done so.

If you want to delay the birth until help arrives, try lying on the floor with your bottom high in the air and your head on your crossed arms on the floor. If there is anyone with you, get them to put on a heater and get a couple of towels ready to wrap the baby in. Put them on a radiator until needed. (The most common reason for transferring babies to hospital is because they have become too cold; they lose heat very rapidly, especially when they are still wet and are in a temperature below 25 degrees Centigrade.)

WHAT TO DO

All you need to do is catch the baby and keep it warm.

- Find something soft on which to give birth, and cover it with a towel if possible.
- When you feel the baby's head coming through your perineum, cup it with your hand.
- Once the head is out, feel for any loops of cord around the neck and bring them forward. The baby's head will probably emerge facing your anus and then rotate to face your thigh.

- Wipe the baby's eyes, nose and mouth free of mucus with a clean hanky or your finger.
- Wait for the next contraction and with it, guide the baby's head down so that the shoulder closest to your front can slide underneath your pubic arch. Once it is free, guide the head upwards towards your abdomen so that the lower shoulder can be freed, and its body will follow.
- Dry the baby with a towel and wrap it in a fresh one. Keep the baby as warm as possible and put it to your breast.
- Do not do anything with the cord.
- The placenta will probably come away within half an hour, especially if you are upright and feeding the baby. If no help has arrived by the time the placenta is delivered, wrap it separately from the baby and keep the two together. Do not attempt to cut or tie the cord.
- Send for help if you have not already done so.

WOMEN'S STORIES

"Even now, some 15 months later, the birth of my second daughter Gwen is very vivid and clear in my mind. Since my first birth experience had been anything but pleasant (having an epidural and a totally managed birth), I was unprepared as to how a natural birth would feel.

"Two weeks before my due date, I had experienced nagging pains, like a period, all weekend. On the Monday I felt very restless but perfectly fit and went to bed as usual that night.

"I woke up about half past one with a slight stomach ache and the 'runs'. I decided to get up and have a bath to relax me, leaving my husband Frank asleep in bed. After a while in the bath, I noticed that my stomach pains were very sharp, short and close together. Since they did not fit the classic wave of labour pains, I assumed that I was not really in labour yet. I got out of the bath and was immediately sick. I thought that something must be happening, so decided to wake Frank up.

"We had recently hired some TENS equipment, so we spent a few minutes looking at the instructions, fitting a new battery, and trying to find glasses and contact lenses, etc. (An object lesson here – test out your equipment before the event.) My pains were no worse and not particularly painful. Frank taped the electrodes to my back and went off to have a shower.

"We both assumed that, as my last labour was some 18 hours long, we would have plenty of time at home until it was time to go into hospital. I looked at my watch; it was two o'clock.

"When Frank came out of the shower, I was bent over the bed breathing hard, I was using the TENS equipment and pressing it for each contraction, but I had not yet turned it up beyond 3 (the dial goes up to 10).

"'Those contractions seem very fast and furious,' Frank observed, 'Have you timed them?'

"'Of course I haven't,' I snapped at him. I felt dreadful, really ratty and bad-tempered. 'I'm going to be sick – get me a bowl.'

"At that moment I realised I had to make another dash to the loo. Frank had been timing my contractions and had decided to phone the hospital. As I went into the bathroom, I caught sight of myself in the mirror – I looked dreadful, as white as a sheet. 'Oh no,' I thought, 'I've got another eight hours of this at least.' I still felt really irritable, though not in any pain – the contractions were still short and sharp, but perfectly bearable, like a gippy tummy.

"As I sat on the loo, I felt the most comfortable I'd been for some time. 'This is better,' I thought, 'maybe I'll stay here.' It was ten past two.

"Suddenly, I felt an enormous churning sensation inside me. At that moment instinct took over and I dropped the TENS equipment and fell on my knees, put my head on the floor and panted as if my life depended on it. I had still not realised what had happened, when Frank came down the corridor. 'The hospital say come in at once,' he said turning into the bathroom, 'Oh my God.'

"With my head on the floor and panting away, I kept thinking 'You must not push against an undilated cervix.' I then put my hand down between my legs. The membranes were bulging out like a balloon, but had not broken. 'What shall I do about this?' I asked, perfectly calmly. 'I'll go and ask them,' and he shot away to have another conversation with the hospital.

"I really felt like two people then. My mind was clear and I was thinking calmly and issuing instructions to Frank – phone Nikki (our nanny), put towels on the floor. It suddenly dawned on me that the baby would be born here, in the bathroom.

"I started to make strange noises and kept trying to kneel upright; while my body was getting on with the process of the birth my mind was concentrating on not pushing – I was determined not to push and risk a tear. By now Frank could see the baby's head; I put my hand down to feel it. I then realised that I was not stretched enough yet – more panting and head on the floor. The effort of not pushing was unbearable. It would be so easy to give in and push.

"Frank told me a midwife was on the way, but since the hospital was some distance away this information did not comfort me in the least. He dashed away to phone again.

"I heard Nikki's key in the door, I knelt upright, and found myself holding the baby's head. 'Help me!' I yelled.

"Frank and Nikki rushed into me. Frank took the baby's head. 'It's all right,' he said, 'I've got it.' There was a pause as the head turned. Instinctively again, I suppose, I stuck my fingers through the membrane and ruptured it. The baby then shot out into Frank's hands. He held the baby face down and pulled all the membranes off it, the baby sneezed and started turning pink. 'Oh look,' I said, 'It's going pink.'

"We had not looked to see, what sex it was. 'A girl,' said Frank, turning her over briefly. Nikki wrapped her in some towels and handed her to me. I looked down at her. A pair of bright blue almond-shaped eyes stared back at me intently – she looked very serious!

"The three of us sat on the floor and stared at each other – we were all as white as sheets. In the next room Sian slept peacefully, unaware of the drama her little sister had caused. I looked at my watch, it was a little after half past two."

Sue Gerryts

"My second daughter is two now. Frankly she has all the delicacy of a bouncing ball, little patience and a personality that announces itself way ahead of her arrival. I should have been prepared for this, alerted by the manner of her birth – sudden, surprising and over before you knew it.

"She was due on Christmas Eve, but about a week earlier I'd felt a bit uncomfortable and popped in to the hospital to check upon things. No chance, said the midwife. This baby's not going to appear this side of Christmas. A few days later I felt a bit 'odd' and called the midwife. We had a chat, she had a feel (not an internal) and she suggested that I looked tired. A hot bath, she said, some painkillers, a hot drink and lots of sleep. Sounded good to me, so we packed daughter number one off to a friend's to play and me into bed. I drifted into and out of sleep, tossed and turned a bit and then realised I was sweating a lot and mumbling. I sometimes mutter and mumble my way through bad periods and this felt the same. So I muttered and tossed and mumbled and turned and just wanted to go to sleep.

"And then I think my waters broke. I say I think because the sensations are all so confused and I might just have wet the bed, but I was certainly suddenly very wet and at precisely the same moment I felt the urge to push. Had I not had a baby before I would have thought I just needed to go to the toilet, and frankly as it was I wasn't 100 per cent sure that that wasn't what it was. Just in case, though, I got on to all fours and began to pant, whilst simultaneously screaming for my partner.

"I explained, as if he didn't know, that I was having a baby. He took one look and rushed off to be somewhere else. He reappeared a few minutes later with his coat on and holding mine. 'Come on', he said, 'we'll go to the hospital.'

"'No, no,' I said, 'I'm having a baby NOW.'

"'Oh God,' he said, and rushed off again. Just in case it wasn't a baby that wanted out, I waddled out into the bathroom and sat on the toilet. Gingerly I reached down for a feel and there was no further doubt about it.

"'See,' I said to my partner when he came back, 'the head's crowning.'

"'They're on their way,' he said. 'Who?' said I. 'Everybody.'

"And then the phone rang. Off he rushed again. I'd been fairly calm until then really; a few groans perhaps, and the odd rude word, but just then I felt the most tremendous urge to push and I got scared and loud at the same time. The baby's head was born to the most tremendous cacophony of screams and swearing, but by the time my partner came back I was able to announce this development quite calmly.

"The next push came almost immediately and Isobel slipped out with barely a gasp.

"He and I were both giggly. I held her to my breast and

checked she was a her and that nothing obvious was wrong. All three of us then sat around stupefied for a while till the phone rang again. It was the flying squad checking on progress. As soon as they heard she'd been born they asked if we were keeping her warm. It was after all, December 21. I decided to try and get back to bed, mess notwithstanding. So, with the cord still between my legs, and hugging Isobel firmly, I did some more of my waddling and got back into bed. We wrapped her in a towel and giggled a bit more.

"The doorbell rang and all of a sudden the room was full of people – ambulancemen, doctors, midwives. It felt like an army of outsiders, but they were all very kind and efficient. Isobel's cord was cut and she was whisked downstairs into the incubator in the ambulance, just to keep her warm, explained the doctor. Usually when they come that fast they're fine. I would have liked to have known that before.

"They decided to leave the placenta where it was, still inside until we got to the hospital. They insisted on carrying me down the stairs, which seemed awkward and unnecessary. In retrospect I was probably not a pretty sight; as I was put into the ambulance you could almost hear the net curtains twitching up and down the road.

"The contractions I had in the ambulance on the way to hospital were the most painful I'd had throughout the whole thing. I had the injection as soon as I arrived and I swear that producing the afterbirth was a more distressing and painful experience than producing the baby. I was, of course, lying down by this time. That over, however, most of the attention switched to the baby. I lay there in a bit of a haze until my partner walked in. He'd stayed behind to see about daughter number one and the mess. I promptly burst into tears and realised that I was in shock. With no rescue remedy to hand we had to make do with that good old British standby, the hot sweet cup of tea.

"The midwife who had visited me earlier had assured me that there was definitely nothing happening. That was about 2.30 pm. I realised that I was about to give birth at about 4.30 pm and Isobel arrived at 4.50 pm. The world and his wife invaded my bedroom about quarter of an hour later.

"I wouldn't say that I'd been in pain at any time. Discomfort, yes, even severe discomfort, but not pain. I was scared, but I didn't even have time to be really frightened. My body took over at half past four and nothing was going to stop it until the baby was born. The me that is separate from my body was almost irrelevant – nothing I wanted or could do would have made the slightest difference. I was functioning as a baby-producing machine. My only wish now is that I'd had a bit more time to enjoy it. As it was, because I hadn't really experienced a 'birth', more a sort of arrival. I didn't really feel as if I'd had my baby properly, and even felt a bit cheated. Now I just feel very proud of myself and my body. And my baby."

Kim Pearl

11 problems in labour

Problems in labour are the big bogey with which women are often threatened when they ask to have their babies at home. Statistically less likely to occur than in hospital, they are none the less a possibility. Although women choosing a home birth may be justifiably more confident about things going smoothly than their medical advisors are, they must, in order to make an informed choice, contemplate the possibility of things going wrong.

You need to think about what might happen, what contingency plans should be made for such an event, what treatment could be given to either you or the baby while still at home and when it would be advisable or necessary to transfer to hospital. You should also be aware of ways of preventing a problem arising if possible, or of helping yourself once it has.

Rates of transfer to hospital while in labour vary wildly. For examples, the NICE draft guidelines[38] on intrapartum care show that transfer rates in labour vary from 32.4 per cent to 56.3 per cent for first time mothers and 1.2 per cent to 17.4 per cent for whom it is not a first baby, with wide regional differences – the highest transfer rates for booked home births both in pregnancy and labour being in the Northern Region, although the figures that they are using are ten or more years old. If it is recommended for you, you should be completely convinced about the need for hospitalisation, because it can be bitterly disappointing even when essential. If you are left with doubts about its necessity, or feel that it was for the benefit of your attendants rather than you or the baby, you can be left with a lingering sense of fury or frustration; Jan's story illustrates this well (see page 172). You may get some clue as to whether this is likely to happen from the prevailing attitude during your antenatal care, although lack of enthusiasm beforehand does not mean that your midwife will not help and encourage you in labour. Most feel that if you are definitely booked for home birth, then it is their professional duty to do their best for you in the circumstances (and in indeed that is endorsed by the March 2006 NMC circular, see page 74). Unfortunately not every midwife sees an encouraging and positive attitude as part of her duty, so that it is as well to be prepared for this. If transfer is suggested and you do not feel convinced that it is necessary, you can ask the following questions:

- What is the indication for transfer?
- What benefit will it have?
- Are there any risks involved in that course of action?
- What alternative treatments are there?
- What will happen if nothing is done?

Of course you are dependent on truthful answers to these questions, and in some situations you may not get them if they are a reflection of the anxiety a midwife feels about home birth. In most instances, however, it will be apparent to you, and you will be grateful for extra help.

Problems arising in labour can be separated into those occurring before and after delivery. The difference is that in most cases problems arising in labour will develop gradually so that there is adequate time for a decision about transfer to be made if necessary. Problems at or after birth tend to manifest themselves suddenly and cause more alarm; it is these emergencies that most concern those opposed to home birth. Taken individually they are as follows.

ANTEPARTUM HAEMORRHAGE

This is bleeding from the vagina before delivery, at any time from 28 weeks on. A little bleeding is not uncommon prior to labour as the mucus plug is lost from the cervix and its changing shape detaches the membranes around it from the uterus. A mucus plug is not always solid; it can also be runny and bloody, but it will probably sit on top of a pad instead of soaking into it. If the bleeding is enough to soak a pad you should call your midwife. It does not necessarily indicate trouble and can occur quite normally, but should be checked. Bleeding also occurs normally and naturally towards the end of labour and this can be regarded as a sign of progress.

However there are two situations where bleeding is a cause for alarm. Both have already been mentioned as they can occur in later pregnancy, but they may also, rarely, show up for the first time in labour. They are placenta abruptio, when the placenta becomes prematurely detached from the uterus, and placenta praevia, when the placenta blocks the exit from the uterus (see also page 104).

It can be difficult to distinguish early cases of placenta abruptio from normal but heavy bleeding at the start of labour. Signs that the placenta might be separating would be a severe, constant abdominal pain over the site of the placenta. The pain does not come and go, unlike contractions. The uterus might remain rock hard instead of relaxing in between contractions, and you would probably have symptoms of shock – feeling faint, cold and clammy, breathless and gasping for air, being thirsty, having spots in front of the eyes or blurred vision, ringing in the ears and generally feeling weak. It is possible that you could have these symptoms with little or no apparent bleeding, because the blood lost was 'concealed' or internal. Either way you should call an ambulance immediately as the baby probably needs to be delivered urgently by Caesarean section in order to stand a chance of survival.

Placenta praevia is unlikely to be revealed for the first time in labour. It would normally give rise to bright red, painless bleeding in pregnancy. It is most unlikely to have gone unnoticed if you have had a scan. However, heavy bleeding should be reported to your midwife immediately. If the bleeding is caused by anything but the most marginal placenta praevia, delivery will need to be by Caesarean section, and even marginal placenta praevia will probably mean delivery in hospital because of the risk of torrential bleeding.

FETAL DISTRESS IN LABOUR

Fetal distress is detected by listening to the baby's heart, generally in between contractions, either with a Pinard stethoscope (the trumpet type) or a portable Sonicaid which uses ultrasound to pick up the baby's heartbeat and can give a digital readout of the rate. It can be amplified so that it can be heard by everyone present.

The baby's heartbeat varies throughout labour, and this is how it should be – a very uniform beat is not necessarily healthy. However, if the baby becomes short of oxygen, perhaps because of the effect of pressure on it, particularly if it is not in an ideal position, if the cord is tight or compressed, or if the placenta is inefficient or deteriorating, its heartbeat can either become much faster or much slower, or becomes very irregular. A fetal heartbeat below 100 beats per minute or above 160 beats per minute can be an indication of oxygen shortage. If the baby's heart was persistently below 100 beats per minute in the first stage of labour, your midwife would probably want you to go into hospital, as this is a sign that the baby is not coping very well with the stress of labour and might need to be delivered rapidly. A heartbeat at this level in the second stage is to be expected, although some midwives might feel that you were better off in hospital.

The baby's heartbeat may also dip or slow in response to contractions. If this happens at the same time as the contraction, known as type 1 dips, it should not give rise to concern. It can be quite usual, especially in transition and second stage, and may well be improved by a change in the mother's position. However type 2 dips (also known as late deceleration) – the slowing of the baby's heart after the contraction is over – is considered to be a sign of distress and, depending how advanced labour is, would raise the question of transfer. If the baby's heart rate drops suddenly when you are in the second stage you would be given an episiotomy and urged to push hard.

Another possible sign of fetal distress is meconium staining of the amniotic fluid or liquor. This is where the baby discharges the contents of its bowels into the fluid that surrounds it. This can only normally be seen when the membranes have ruptured. Meconium can either be greeny-black, which indicates that it has been passed recently and might indicate current distress, or it might be golden-brown, which can mean it has been passed some time ago and indicates distress in the past. Fresh meconium, especially if it is thick or tenacious or if the liquor contains lumps of meconium, is the more worrying, although it is thought that only 25 per cent of babies with meconium staining are actually short of oxygen.[39] If fresh meconium staining was accompanied by irregularities in the baby's heartbeat it would be advisable to go into hospital unless the birth was imminent. Midwives are under instruction to take women with meconium staining into hospital, although the NICE draft guidelines

(June 2006) state that lightly meconium stained liquor does not indicate transfer to a consultant unit from home.

It is important that you feel you can trust your midwife as you have to take her word on the heart rate, unless she uses a Sonicaid or you get your partner to listen. Trust your instincts – subjective signs of distress include the baby moving frantically or moving very much less, although babies commonly move little in labour.

How you can help yourself

If the baby is showing signs of distress, try moving your position frequently. Do not lie on your back; if you are standing, try lying on your side; or try all fours or squatting and keep changing it. It may be that in some positions there is a slight pinching of the cord which may be relieved by shifting the baby's position and easing the pressure. You can also ask to be given oxygen from a mask.

LACK OF PROGRESS

This is defined as a failure of the cervix to dilate beyond a certain point, as a failure of the presenting part to descend, or as a failure of the woman to give birth after being in labour for a specified number of hours. Its only cause should be cephalo-pelvic dispro-portion (where the baby's head is too large for your pelvis) but is more commonly due to tension, of which you may not conscious-ly be aware, preventing you from dilating.

This is unlikely to happen at home, where women are more like-ly to be allowed to labour for as long as necessary without arbi-trary time limits set upon the length of their labour. The only sit-uation where home is not likely to be less inhibiting than hospital is where you have someone present who is clearly anxious or dis-approving. If your labour is very slow or stops for this reason (and many women who have their babies at home report this phenom-enon in the presence of visitors), you must ask them to leave. Clearly this can be difficult, but it is more important that your labour progresses satisfactorily than that other people's feelings are protected, even if that person is your midwife or your partner. In fact a skilled and sensitive midwife should be able to see when this is happening and facilitate a change.

If it is the midwife who is causing the problem through her attitude, then you must ask for a change, or at least ask her to stay in another room until called. You have the right to ask for any midwife to be changed if you are not getting on well. This applies in advance, so that if, during your antenatal care, you encounter a midwife that you feel certain you would not want in labour, write to the local midwifery supervisor and request that this particular midwife is not sent to you when you are in labour. You do not have to give a reason, but it will help the supervisor to improve the service if you tell her of anything that this midwife has done or said to you that you feel is unprofessional. Sometimes it will be what she does not say or do, she may just be very unenthusiastic and it is as well to protect yourself from such negativity beforehand. The option of changing the midwife may not be open to women living in very isolated areas or where units are short-staffed, but it is none the less worth expressing your feelings. If you are having good contractions and feel relaxed, and yet labour is not progressing, there may be some disproportion, although it is unlikely if it is not your first baby. If the baby is not distressed, try squatting (see also following page, posterior babies). If there is true failure to progress and the baby is in distress, you will need to be delivered in hospital, perhaps with forceps, ventouse or by Caesarean. However it is quite possible for labour that is allowed to take its own course to last over 40 hours (not all of this will be very painful) and, although this is exhausting, you may prefer it to a hospital delivery. In this situation you need lots of encouragement, good food and as much rest as you can get. Sometimes contractions cease so that you can get some sleep and then begin again later.

How you can help yourself

Progress can sometimes be made by changing your position, preferably to an upright one. It can sometimes be very tempting to stay in a position which does not hurt too much, and it may require courage to adopt a position which brings on stronger, more effective contractions. Try also drinking raspberry leaf tea. If you know you are feeling tense, a glass of wine or beer might help; do not have much, though, because alcohol can inhibit uterine contractions. Massage may help; and you should visualise your cervix opening and keep saying 'Open' to yourself. Nipple rolling or stimulation will produce the hormone oxytocin, which will boost your contractions and encourage labour. It might also help to have a long, deep bath. Try plugging the overflow with plasticine to make it deeper. Get someone to apply firm pressure to the balls of your feet. Homeopathic remedies include Pulsatilla, for contractions which are changeable, with slow dilation when you are tearful. Try Gelsemium for 'false pains', if you are tiring or slowing down. If contractions stop, take Caulophyllum 6 every 15 minutes (Caulophyllum is not recommended in pregnancy unless a definite need for it has been demonstrated).

If you want to check your own progress in labour you can do your own vaginal examination (this is easier if you are already familiar with the feel of your cervix). First wash your hands thoroughly and then reach into your vagina with one or two fingers. You are unlikely to be in advanced labour if you cannot feel your cervix, because it descends and becomes more accessible as labour is established. As it progresses the head comes down and the cervix becomes lower. The cervix is gradually effaced or taken up into the body of the uterus, so that eventually all that remains is the tissue stretched over the head. It might feel like something slimy over a grapefruit, or you may feel the membranes like taut cling-film with the amniotic fluid behind them. The hole left by the dilating cervix is completely round, and when you are fully dilated there is no rim left at all. You can check your dilatation by estimating how many fingers you could get into the hole; one finger is equal to 2 cm, two fingers is equal to 3.5 cm, three fingers to 5.5 cm, four to 7.5 cm. Full dilation is when there is no rim and the hole measures 10 cm. Remember, the cervix can dilate very suddenly in a short time.

MALPOSITION OF THE BABY

Persistent malpositions should have been detected in pregnancy, but the baby may alter its position at the last minute or you may want to have the baby at home despite its position. Try taking homeopathic Pulsatilla 200 for all malpositions.

Occiput posterior (OP or POP)

This is where the baby's back is against your back, instead of against the abdominal wall which is the more common and more favourable position. You may be able to tell that your baby is posterior if you feel the kicks at the front or if there is a saucer-like dip around your navel. If the head fails to engage before labour, especially with a first baby, it may be posterior. If you know this before labour starts you should try and alter its position by spending a lot of time on all fours. It is thought that gravity helps the heaviest part of the head, the back, to swing round so that the baby faces your back (occiput anterior, OA).

If the baby becomes posterior in labour, spend as much time as you can on all fours; in most cases (80 per cent) babies rotate spontaneously during labour, but this can help. Posterior labours tend to be longer, and perhaps more painful; they are often accompanied by a lot of backache. If you can cope with the pain, and progress is being made, there should be no reason to transfer you. If the baby remains in a posterior position you may experience a premature urge to push, and the baby may be born face to pubes. Squatting should help the baby out, but because of the position of the head its diameters will be larger than otherwise and progress may be delayed in the second stage. An episiotomy may be necessary. If you are unable to push the baby out you will have to be transferred to hospital for an instrumental delivery. Five per cent of babies who start off OP fail to rotate either to an anterior or posterior position and get their heads stuck diagonally across the pelvis in a transverse arrest. This is rare but, if the baby does not rotate, rotational forceps (Kielland's) will be required in order to deliver it. If the second stage is delayed but progress is being made, although slowly, and the baby is not distressed, then you should be allowed to push for as long as you can.

Shoulder presentation/transverse lie

If your baby lies across your abdomen and cannot be persuaded to change its position, it cannot be born at home. This may also apply if it keeps changing its position. The baby can be persuaded to turn head down, or it might be helped into this position while your membranes are ruptured (known as a stabilising induction). If it will not budge, though, delivery has to be by Caesarean section. You may prefer to wait until you go into spontaneous labour to see if this will be necessary; some of the reports in this book record last minute changes of position.

Face and brow presentation

If the baby deflexes or extends its head in labour so that it is not curved into a ball, it can make things difficult because the diameters of its face or brow are wider than the back of the head. Such a baby can alter its position in labour but, if it does not, delivery may have to be by Caesarean section.

PROBLEMS AT THE TIME OF DELIVERY

Shoulder dystocia

This is a real problem which arises when a baby's shoulders become stuck after its head is delivered. This is more common with larger babies. Very interestingly, two studies used in the NICE intrapartum draft guidelines, from Australia and the U.S., show a lower incidence of shoulder dystocia in home births.[40]

The orthodox way of treating it is to put the mother on her back with her legs in stirrups and to use force to pull the baby out. Another solution is for the woman to lie on her back and bring her knees up to her chest which can have the effect of straightening the birth canal. She can also try squatting, opening her pelvis to its maximum and leaning on her abdomen to exert leverage on the baby, although this is said to increase the risk of uterine rupture. If all these methods were to fail then the attendant has to break the baby's clavicle to decrease the width of the shoulders. Time is limited in this situation because, once the head is out, the placental site becomes smaller and starts to separate. The baby cannot expand its chest and breathe so it is deprived of oxygen.

If your baby's shoulders become stuck when you are delivering at home, the best thing to do seems to be to turn on to all fours. Ina May Gaskin has produced some convincing evidence that suggests that this is the least damaging and most successful way of treating the problem; she says that 'sometimes the baby who seemed to be tightly wedged with the mother in semi-recumbent position will virtually fall out once the mother is on hands and knees'.[41] As your midwife may be unfamiliar with this, it might be up to you to take this action as soon as it becomes clear what the problem is. It is less likely to occur if you are delivering in a squatting position. It is interesting that shoulder dystocia is not usually used to scare women away from choosing home birth because hospitals cannot offer any advantage in this situation.

WOMEN'S STORIES

A midwife who is practised at delivering babies at home, and who feels that it is undoubtedly the best place to be born, told me of two occasions where it seemed as though the mothers intuitively knew that things were going to go wrong and that they should go into hospital despite their original decisions to have their babies at home. She feels that if you choose a hospital birth you give up any idea of the birth being your responsibility and don't believe anything your body is telling you. If you are booked for home, it is your responsibility and you are much more acutely aware of yourself. It does seem as though you can have an instinct about your labour or birth which it is wise to heed – either one way or the other.

The first mother was booked for a domino on the understanding that if all went well she would have the baby at home. She had reached 3-4 cm without any difficulty. The baby's heartbeat was fine and there was no indication of any problem when the mother said, 'I've got to go in, I know something is going to go wrong.' The midwife was quite disappointed as she was anticipating a happy home birth, but they went in and the mother reached 9 cm without any problems. However, she stuck at this dilatation for the next 3 hours. It turned out that the baby was presenting with his head on one side, a position that isn't even recognised in obstetrics. The registrar attempted to push him back up and alter his position, but half an hour later the mother was being prepared for Caesarean section which she was begging the staff to perform. The registrar repeated the manual manoeuvre, putting his whole hand into her vagina and urging her to push. She pushed hard and the baby was born normally, although he was taken to the special care nursery as there were fears that he might have sustained a cerebral haemorrhage. Fortunately this was not the case.

The second incident concerned a woman who was booked to have her baby at home. She too had reached 3-4 cm when she said 'something is going to go wrong'. They went into the hospital together and the mother had a massive postpartum haemorrhage requiring a lot of resuscitation.

"I changed my hospital booking after hearing a midwife talk about how women needed less pain relief at home, and I thought it sounded good and Adrian agreed.

"I went into labour two weeks early, starting with a strange pain every 12 minutes. I rang Adrian who had just got to Kent, he came back and we had friends round for coffee – my neighbour brought me flowers and sandwiches, and we went shopping in Tesco's.

"At 4.00 the contractions were more powerful and we called the midwife, and she arrived with her assistant. We cleared the nursery and put waterproof sheeting down. We sat around drinking tea; my mum and sister arrived. As it got more painful Adrian and I went up to the nursery to be on our own. My mum said she could hear me laughing in between contractions!

"By 9.00, Isobel, our midwife, found I was 7 cm and she told Adrian the baby would be here in time for last orders!

"By 10.30 I wanted to start pushing and tried every possible position – on the toilet, squatting, standing, on all-fours, on my front, on my back . . . but I couldn't push the baby out. A second midwife came to help but by 12.00 midnight still nothing had happened and I was very despondent. My blood pressure was very high and Isobel said that if nothing had happened by 12.30 we would have to go in. I was exhausted.

"Eventually they made a 999 call and I walked to the ambulance, trying not to push. I had two gasps of gas and air in the ambulance but I kept losing it – it was a horrible feeling. Unbeknown to me my mother and sister were following.

"We finally got in, and it was scary at this point. The surgeon came and gave me an internal and agreed forceps were needed. I felt really scared when they were putting in the epidural and I had to do without the TENS machine. Adrian was completely ashen. It was wonderful once it took effect though, I was back to me again and my Mum and sister were able to come in.

"The surgeon came in and I could virtually feel the contractions so I panted her out with the forceps. She was born at 2.35 am and weighed 6 lb 10 oz. Adrian cut the cord and then she fed straightaway for two hours.

"Initially I was disappointed – I had enjoyed being at home with my family and friends around me, and not felt nervous or scared of the consequences there. The hospital was noisy and intrusive although the staff were brilliant. But Isobel said that I had done so well just on the TENS machine, and I had been able to try pushing her out for far longer than I would have been allowed in hospital, and that took the disappointment away. It would have been silly to insist on staying at home if it meant threatening my life or Amelia's."

Alison Smith

"I was booked to have my first baby at home and had a pool for a water birth when I went into labour properly at 12 on Sunday night.

"At 5.30 in the morning the first midwife called. I'd had the TENS on for about an hour then. She checked me and found that I was 2-3 cm dilated and advised me to carry on walking round and feeling comfortable at home and she would come back at lunchtime. I had Steve, my husband, and his mother with me, and I felt happy with that. I had the midwife's bleep number in case I needed her in a hurry, and at 5.00 pm she checked me again. This time I was 5 cm. She left and came back at 9.00 pm when she decided to stay as I was wondering whether to get into the pool. They like you to wait until you are 5 cm dilated otherwise contractions can slow down.

"I was still happy watching the telly, going to the loo and being sick.

"Joan, the midwife, was the one I was booked with. Luckily she was on duty. I had a nice relationship with her and I never felt pressurised by her. At about 12.00 the second midwife was called because they thought I would have had the baby by the morning, because the contractions were quite strong.

"I got into the pool then and stayed there, although I had to get out every hour to go to the toilet. It was only then that I realised how effective the pool was at relieving pain. The toilet is upstairs and the pool was downstairs, and I found myself running downstairs to get back into the pool.

"At 4.00 am I was no further dilated and we agreed that the midwives should rupture my membranes. I was starting to get tired, contractions were still quite regular – every 3 minutes – but I was still only 6 cm. I was still being sick quite often, although I was able to continue eating and drinking.

"At 6.30 am I got out of the pool again, still no further dilated, although contractions were really strong and the midwives thought I was going to deliver soon.

"I think they were getting a bit worried although they didn't force me to go in, because the baby was okay. They gave me the option of pethidine to give me a break, but I was against that because I didn't want the baby born drugged up, although by this time I was absolutely exhausted.

"Eventually Joan said, 'Do you want to go in? If you do, I'll come with you.' She was really supportive, and by this time I was getting worried myself, so we decided to go in, although I was quite upset about it as I had everything all sorted out at home.

"So I had to get out and get dressed which I found distressing because I was shaking and had no pain relief. Fortunately, I had packed a bag so I didn't have to hunt around for things – and so we went in – Steve's mother driving us, with Joan following behind.

"I was relieved to get there and have the baby monitored and discover that it was all right. Once that was done, we examined my options – they offered to put up a Syntocinon drip because I had been at 6 cm for 12 hours. Once I had agreed to that, I accepted an epidural and the anaesthetist was very good about explaining, and gave me a mobile epidural which gave me a new lease of life, and meant I was still able to wander about with the community midwives.

"By the evening though there were no community staff left – they were exhausted too, so I was handed over to the hospital staff, which was disappointing but understandable.

"Then there was some confusion because the registrar thought I was fully dilated and suggested the epidural was allowed to wear off, and then the midwife found I was still only 7 cm, so it was topped up again. An hour later the consultant felt I was 9 cm and sent Steve and my mother-in-law home for a rest. In fact, I was still only 7 cm and she said that we would have to get the baby out by 10 pm. They topped up the epidural again – I was shattered – and I had a wash and tried to sleep.

"All of a sudden, the baby got really distressed and within ten minutes I had been shaved, signed the consent form and was down the corridor having a Caesarean under general anaesthetic. Unfortunately the epidural could not be topped up in time, and at 10.15 pm James was born weighing 7 lb 13 oz.

"Steve and my mother-in-law stayed with me from then on, but I was so exhausted that I did not come round until 2 am on Wednesday evening.

"I do regret that everyone else saw him before me and wish that the Caesarean could have been under epidural. But James is healthy and despite the start I was able to breastfeed him successfully. I was given a lot of support and encouragement over that, and now he won't even take a bottle.

"I'm sure I was given more time at home than I would have been in hospital. Nobody knows why I didn't dilate fully and I'll have a trial of labour next time."

Jackie Mayne

"I was expecting to have my second baby at home. I had no trouble booking it, as I live in an area where home birth is considered a normal option, and the midwives emphasised that there would be no difficulty if I decided in labour that I wanted to go in after all.

"I was quite tired at the outset of labour but it started well with contractions coming every two minutes right from the start. After 5 hours they were coming every minute and a half and I was getting exhausted. However this went on for another seven hours, by which time I was fully dilated but had no urge to push whatsoever. The baby's head was still very high and I was absolutely knackered. I asked to go into hospital, and although the midwife agreed to call the ambulance, I felt she was not keen on my taking this decision. (I later discovered that although she had attended lots of home births she had never had to transfer anyone.) She kept on urging me to push and when the ambulance arrived I heard her say to the driver 'she only pushed for half an hour'.

"I had heard that women who were booked for home and had to transfer were likely to receive a hostile reception at the hospital but this turned out to be untrue. The medical staff were very kind and helpful and took pains to explain what was going on. While they were out of the room the midwife continued to urge me to push and seemed not to understand that I couldn't.

One of the other midwives urged me on by saying another woman there had been pushing for three hours.

"The anaesthetist set up an epidural in order for the baby to be delivered by ventouse. We had been there 25 minutes when the baby's heartbeat showed signs of great distress – it stopped beating with every contraction, and I was given oxygen. The room suddenly filled with doctors and my son was delivered by ventouse very rapidly. I was very glad that I was in hospital at this point and wonder if an inner instinct had told me that this was what I needed to do.

"I feel that if you accept responsibility for your birth as you do if you choose birth at home, then it should be recognised that you are the one that makes the decisions and that they should be supported, even when that decision involves going into hospital."

Sally Smith

"I was expecting the birth of my third child to be quite quick as the first had been seven hours following induction and my daughter's birth only took five hours. I went into spontaneous labour at about two in the morning when I was four days over-due, and at this time I thought the baby would be born by breakfast-time. We called the midwife out straightaway, but nothing much seemed to be happening so she left, to return at 6.00 am.

"By this time I was in strong labour, had reached 6 cm and was using the TENS machine. I took it off to get in the bath, and I would have liked to stay there longer but there wasn't room for both my husband and the midwife in there together.

"By lunchtime there was still no baby although my daughter had been ringing from school at every break to see if it had arrived. Eventually I reached the second stage and started to push. I remember finding it very hard work – it lasted two hours. When the head finally emerged, I thought thank God for that, it's over! But then the room suddenly went very quiet and everyone started saying 'push, push some more!'

"It was evident that his shoulders were stuck and I remem-ber everyone panicking and the midwife's assistant on the phone calling an ambulance. Fortunately I had been on all fours for all of the second stage [the best position for shoulder dystocia, see page 161] and my midwife who has very small hands was able to reach in under his arm and pull him out. Ben was not in wonderful condition, he was blue with the cord round his neck which terrified my husband. He needed oxygen, his Apgar score was around the middle range, but they cancelled the ambulance.

"The midwives had given me Syntometrine thinking that I was likely to haemorrhage after having a big baby and consequently I had a retained placenta. Everything clamped down and they called the paramedics to help. However after two hours the Syntometrine had worn off and I had enough energy to give a couple more pushes and push it out, so I was able to send the paramedics away.

"Ben weighed 12 lbs – at least. That was the maximum weight the scales went up to and he tipped that so he may have weighed more. I think the midwife almost left the profession after his birth; she was in quite a state about it for a while as it was her first case of shoulder dystocia.

"Later she felt glad that she had met the challenge. Ben did have a 'waiter's tip' palsy to start with and we had to take him to hospital to be X-rayed to see if his collarbone was broken. However, within a couple of days he was fine and there is no long-term damage."

Jan Hibbert

"When I was expecting my first baby, I initially asked for a home birth. I was persuaded out of it by stories of what could go wrong, although nobody told me about what could go wrong in hospital, so I decided on a domino. In fact they said they weren't available for first-time mothers so I asked for home again and got the domino.

"As time went on, and I visited the home birth support group, I became more confident and asked for a home birth again. They were very reluctant, citing my shoe size – 3 – as being against me, but they went along with it, although I feel now that they never had any intention of delivering me at home.

"When I went into labour we called the midwife, whose attitude was negative from the outset. When I wanted to eat scrambled egg on toast, she said, 'You can't be in labour if you want to eat that!' She discouraged me from walking about, preferring that I sat down, and prevented me from going out with Tony and the dog for a walk.

"She examined me, said I was 'only' 3 cm, and without asking me, did an excruciating sweep of membranes. She said that my membranes were tough as old boots and that she had failed to rupture them with a little finger stall that she had put on and which people didn't usually notice because it was so small. I did not feel sufficiently confident to tell her to get out, which is what I should have done.

"Eventually, like fools, we did let her rupture the membranes and there was meconium in the liquor. At this point, the midwife said we must go in or we would have a dead or damaged baby. She said the baby's heartbeat was irregular (although reading the notes later, this did not appear to be true). When we got there she claimed there was not enough room for the baby to come down, in direct contrast to what she had told us earlier.

"I asked to come off the monitor but the doctor said the trace showed the baby was sleepy – he then offered pethidine which I refused saying it would make the baby more sleepy. He then wanted to accelerate labour, which I objected to saying it would make labour more painful. He replied, 'Labour is painful, what do you expect?'

"I was offered an epidural and I said this would increase the chance of my having forceps and episiotomy – he said 'this was rubbish'. I'm sure I was labelled the 'failed home birth' and everything that happened to me including the fetal blood sampling contributed to making me feel as though I was being punished for wanting to have a home birth. I felt as though I couldn't perform in hospital and after being confined to bed, with acceleration of labour and an epidural (after the midwife telling me I would be hours and hours yet) the baby became distressed and I eventually had a Caesarean section under epidural. The whole thing was a nightmare.

"I would say to anyone who is having a home birth and might be transferred – have someone with you. We chose not to because we felt we wanted it to be a private affair and we ended up with a football match theatreful. The balance of power would be different if you had someone else there for you.

"Robert will be my only child. I could not go through that again."

Kate Smith

"I was eight days overdue and concerned about induction when my midwife came round one morning and found I was 2 cm dilated and fully effaced, so she thought it would not be long. I went for a brisk two mile walk and had lots of Braxton Hicks contractions but it all faded away once I got home.

"However, when we were having supper that night I felt a bit sick, and then contractions started about 9.15, with a slight trickle of waters and a show. We thought 'whoopee' and started crushing ice-cubes, getting things ready. The contractions were coming every 3-5 minutes and lasting a minute. The duty midwife found I was 2-3 cm and suggested taking a couple of paracetomol and trying to sleep. I had a bath with plastic sheeting over it to keep the heat in, with candles and soft music playing and I was able to doze a bit.

"At 4.30 am things started hotting up a bit and we called Donna, my midwife, and Louise, a friend who was going to be with us for the birth. By 6.30 I was 5-6 cm dilated, the waters went and I was using the TENS machine and feeling rested and in control.

"At 8.00 I was 7 cm, quite enjoying it, using Entonox. The pain was manageable although it felt as though it was going on a long time. It was all very relaxed and calm, at one point Louise said I wasn't making enough noise! Everyone sat around and let me get on with it. I was hanging over the end of the bed and leaning against Martin most of the time; I didn't walk around much. I was able to keep in touch by staring into Louise's eyes. She was there to hang on to, she was the only one in the room who had had a baby; it added another dimension.

"By 10.00 am I was fully dilated, contractions quietened down and almost nothing happened for half an hour. I was cracking jokes and didn't feel any urge to push. At 10.30 everything switched back on again. I did feel an urge to push but it wasn't overwhelming and it was quite hard work. It felt as though there was something enormous inside that wasn't going to shift. I was propped up against the chest of drawers, and I was able to see her head coming down in the mirror doors opposite, which was a great encouragement. I couldn't believe it was really going to happen but Donna said, 'Look I'm getting ready to deliver a baby.'

"I finally gave one big heave and suddenly saw this enormous mottley-blue thing shoot out. She seemed such a big baby all slithery and bluey-grey. I said, 'What is it?' Nobody answered but they held her up so I could see, and I said, 'Oh it's a girl, it's a girl. It's Holly.' I had a feeling of absolute relief and said, 'She's here, she's arrived!'

"They wrapped her up in a bit of blue cloth and I held her, with her wise, little face looking up at me wide-eyed. She was heavy, 9 lb 6 oz, and I tore a bit with the delivery of the shoulders. Donna thought I might have to go to hospital to be sutured, but once I was cleaned up it didn't seem that bad so she sutured me there.

"There was a great air of celebration: we had champagne and then Holly and I had a lukewarm bath. When we got out the midwives had made the bed up with fresh, clean sheets and then they disappeared leaving Holly, Martin and me together."

Joanne Nicholds

"On 10 August at 12.02 am I gave birth to a beautiful 7 lb daughter, two weeks earlier than expected. It took 20 hours from start to finish and was everything I hoped such an experience should be. Rachel spent her first night sleeping on her father's chest, all three of us together. The midwives felt sure an attempt would have been made to turn her as she was in a persistently occiput posterior position as she began to descend but she rotated naturally as she descended. It was the first home delivery one of them had attended and the second for the other. They were both very favourably impressed and with more support would like to do more."

Jackie Reay

"Our second daughter was born at home at 3.05 am on a Thursday morning. Having fought all our battles to have our first baby at home, my second pregnancy was very peaceful. I believe my antenatal care to have been ideal for a normal pregnancy. All my antenatal appointments except one were with one of the midwives who delivered Rachel (including the booking appointment). The exception was an appointment with a consultant at 28 weeks.

"By contrast the birth was not as straightforward. Sarah was in a posterior position as Rachel had been, but did not turn. Although I did not suffer the classic symptom of severe backache, and I do not recall the pain as being any worse than with Rachel, I seemed unable to push Sarah out. We tried all sorts of positions, and eventually a supported squat brought her head into view, but she then stuck on my perineum. Then quite suddenly she began to show signs of distress when her heartbeat dropped and an episiotomy was performed to deliver her quickly. She breathed immediately and was 'class A' in spite of her difficult time.

"John woke Rachel (now two and a half) immediately and I shall never forget her look of wide-eyed delight at the small slippery person lying on my tummy. Rachel and I looked at the placenta with a student midwife who had come as an observer while we waited for my GP to come and repair the episiotomy. After he had finished we all had tea and toast and, as there were now eight of us (two midwives, one student, one GP and our family, now four), quite a party spirit arose. Then I had a bath, fed Sarah who took to the breast like a veteran, our midwives went home and we went to bed for what was left of the night.

"In retrospect there are a few outstanding reasons why I was glad to have been at home, in spite of some anxious moments. My labour was not augmented with a Syntocinon drip and Sarah was not delivered with forceps, which may well have been the case in hospital. I received no pain relief other than Entonox which meant that I was fully aware of what was happening. My GP did an excellent repair to my perineum which healed rapidly with a minimum of discomfort, and these reasons are all additional to those which had made me determined to have my children born at home."

Jackie Reay

"For some time Nick and I had discussed the idea of a home birth. We wanted to be in familiar surroundings, retain as much control as possible and most importantly to be together during and after the birth. At 35 years of age, pregnant with our first child, I knew that it would be difficult to obtain the cooperation necessary for a home birth. I wanted to enjoy the pregnancy and didn't want to become involved in too much of a tussle with the medical profession. I was certain that I did not want a 'run of the mill' hospital birth.

"From what I had heard, the domino system seemed to be a suitable alternative. The consultant agreed to my request for a domino delivery but, to my disappointment, the district midwives refused. This left only one viable alternative – a home birth. To our surprise, the midwives accepted our request for a home birth without question. So, paradoxically, we were precipitated into our first choice (a home birth) by the unexpected attitude of the district midwives. Later discussion revealed that a home birth was considered to be less demanding on limited resources (under the domino system in our area the district midwife attends the home antenatal visits only, the labour being assigned to the duty midwife).

"I was allocated a midwife, developed a good relationship with her during my pregnancy, and would have been happy to have had her help during my labour. It was disheartening to learn that I had only a one in twelve chance of going into labour while she was on duty. It was during the antenatal home visits that I began to detect that there was little or no real commitment amongst the midwives to the idea of a home birth. I discovered that many of the district midwives have no first-hand experience of a home birth, either during their training or whilst working on the district. The midwife who attended my labour (a complete stranger) greeted me on the doorstep with the remark 'I hoped you wouldn't go into labour this evening, I have never attended a home birth.' She was obviously very nervous about attending a birth outside the hospital environment.

"From comments that were made by the four district midwives that I met before and after the birth of our child, it would appear that a large percentage of women hoping to have their children at home are transferred to hospital during labour. In my case, it might well be that the decision to transfer was taken on entirely legitimate medical grounds. Certainly I had a very good relationship with my GP, found her very supportive and trusted her judgment. However, the decision not to proceed at home seemed to me to be largely influenced by the attitude of the district midwife, who was, from the outset, extremely lacking in confidence. At the time this left me doubting the validity of the decision, frustrated and distressed.

"With hindsight, I suspect that the midwives agreed so readily to a home birth in the hope that I would back down or, failing that, be pressurised at some stage during labour into accepting a transfer to hospital. It seems unlikely that midwives will have the confidence to continue in the home environment with anything other than a short and entirely straightforward labour. If home birth is really on offer, is it not irresponsible of the medical authorities to expect midwives to attend without ensuring that they have the necessary training and experience? If district midwives are not gaining practical experience of home births during their training, it seems to be building a fundamental lack of confidence into the system. I suspect that in most cases, possibly mine included, agreement to provide support for a home birth is nothing more than a gesture.

"Our experience has left us feeling that what we wanted is probably not available through the NHS though we feel strongly that it should be. Next time round we will be looking for more solid support. I can now appreciate why women turn to the expensive services of a private midwife.

"In hospital we found the staff on the labour ward, particularly the midwives, to be considerate, attentive and eager to involve us in the decision making (contrary to our initial prejudices). However, we did feel that the attitude of the staff was, in part, predisposed by their knowledge that we had originally rejected a hospital booking. This, combined with the fact that we had already spent 12 hours at home in labour, forestalled any tendency there might have been on their part to assume control.

"Despite their willingness to accommodate our wishes, the underlying atmosphere was often one of imminent crisis. This resulted in the baby having a fetal monitor, which I later felt to have been unnecessary and would, without the intervention of a senior doctor, almost certainly have led to my having a Caesarean section.

"Happily I can say, without hesitation, that the intense exhilaration I felt at the moment of birth was in no way lessened by being in hospital. However, if I had had to stay in hospital after the birth, in cramped conditions, with no privacy, separated from my husband and subjected to endless routines, I would certainly have hated it.

"Here is a brief account of the labour:

"5 pm. Waters broke, no contractions. Fitted TENS machine in place and spent a couple of hours relaxing with Nick.

"8 pm. Called midwife. Disappointed, when she arrived, to see a stranger. 2 cm dilated. Mild contractions.

"12 pm. Nick and I carried on as we had planned. The midwife seemed to feel very much on the edge of things, though we would have been happy to include her. She decides to sit in another room and come in from time to time.

"2 am. Feeling positive. 6 cm dilated. Contractions much stronger but easier to manage.

"8 am. Contractions very close together but still manageable. Feeling good. Still 6 cm dilated. Midwife is not happy and decides to call in GP. GP arrives within minutes. Examination shows baby is posterior. A long labour is anticipated and midwife is not happy about continuing at home. GP advises that we transfer to hospital. I thought things were going so well. I am very disappointed and in floods of tears.

"9 am. Admitted to hospital. Labour ward sister attentive but irritated. Talks to us with studied patience about 'NCT people'. We are all viewing each other with caution. A bean bag is produced and we continue as at home.

"4 pm. Still only 7 cm dilated. Cervix swollen. Talk of pelvis being wrong shape for normal delivery. Constant talk of Caesarean section. Agree to fetal monitor being attached to baby's head; had felt very opposed to this but find any talk of danger to the baby impossible to resist.

"5 pm. Pushing contractions start. Still 7 cm dilated. Mustn't push. Don't seem to be getting anywhere. Starting to feel low. We are both exhausted. Asked to consider pain relief. Decide on epidural as I am worried by talk of Caesarean. We feel they may suddenly decide this is necessary and I want to make sure I am conscious (up until now I have managed with the TENS and gas and air). Baby in distress scare – doctor thinks I should have Caesarean. Senior doctor called in; he agrees I can continue a bit longer.

"9 pm. Doctors discuss Caesarean with us. Examination

reveals I am almost fully dilated. Doctor suggests we wait for epidural to wear off and try pushing.

"11 pm. Feeling exhausted, want to tell everyone to get lost. Nick and midwife do a great job to get me back into gear. At last I have a purpose again – I push for all I'm worth.

"11.30 pm. Our daughter is born. The midwife prevents the doctor from passing her straight to the waiting paediatrician and she is placed on my tummy. She is alert, peaceful and showing no signs of distress. A brief check (in the same room) and she is back in my arms, suckling at my breast. I feel ecstatic and full of energy.

"1 am. We are taken to a side room for the night. It is wonderful to be alone together for the first time with our daughter.

"10 am. We are discharged and take her home."

Jan Rumball

"I would just like to encourage any mother-to-be to consider a home birth. I have had two out of three children at home and enjoyed the experience very much. With the last baby it was very much touch and go as to whether he would eventually be born at home. Six weeks before he was born he was in the breech position and I was told that I would have a forceps delivery and that I could not have him at home. I was convinced that the baby would turn in time and he did. My waters broke two weeks after he was due, so we called the midwife. When she arrived everything stopped! I was allowed 12 hours, by which time if labour had not started again I would have to go into hospital. Twelve hours came and went and no signs of labour. I had a local doctor who came to tell me I must go into hospital, but my husband and I refused. I was determined to have the baby at home. My husband had to write a letter taking full responsibility. The older midwives were marvellous and very patient with me. Jonathan eventually arrived three days after my waters had broken. They were the longest days of my life! There was no infection on the baby or myself and he arrived in four hours once labour started properly. It is possible to go for four days once the waters have broken, provided you remain indoors, but the midwives of today are not taught this; it is a pity. I would still have had Jonathan at home despite all the problems we came up against, but I could not have done it without my husband's support and strength behind me. He was with me all the way. Having a baby at home is lovely, with all the family around you giving you love and comfort."

Linda Riley

"As soon as I had decided to continue with my IUD failure first pregnancy I knew I wanted a home birth. At home I would have the benefits of continuity of care from my midwives and feel more relaxed and confident in my own surroundings. I felt that many problems that had occurred at hospital were due to a hospital being an institution which is unable to allow for the individual – things are done 'just in case'. At home I could say what I want and be the centre of an event which was irreversibly going to bring enormous changes into my and my husband's life. I accepted the risks of birth and felt the benefits outweighed them. I was also 10 minutes from a large teaching hospital with a special care baby unit.

"I didn't have much difficulty finding a home birth GP. He was dubious as I was a 'first timer', but I had prepared a list of his objections and told him I accepted and knew the possible risks. He agreed as long as everything was entirely normal and I swore I would have Syntometrine in the third stage. My job as counsellor for Brook helped.

"I did feel a pressure to not have any sugar in my urine, etc., which was an additional and unnecessary anxiety.

"From 28 weeks my midwife visited me at home, which was fun and helped me to get to know her. She told me that none of her first time mothers had managed to have their babies at home but had had to be transferred. This strengthened my resolve to be the first.

"Before the birth I wanted a midwife, GP and friends and relatives to be positive. However, doctor colleagues at work said 'How brave, having a home birth', and even my husband would not have opted for home birth. My mother said nothing, but I knew she would have felt safer if I'd have been in hospital.

"In the last weeks the midwife insisted on raising the bed by nine inches – eventually she came by with bed blocks for me. But at this time I didn't think I would get on the bed at all.

"My labour started at 39 weeks at 3.00 am, after I had finished varnishing the kitchen floor the night before. I woke up with period-like pains every five minutes for 50 seconds and my waters leaked gently throughout the labour. It was a beautiful sunny dawn and I went out and walked in the garden before waking my husband. I had a bath while he sat perched on a chair having his breakfast and chatting.

"I helped take a clothes rack out of my room and put my shoes in a bag in between stopping and leaning over furniture whilst having a contraction. By 7.30 am my husband wanted to ring the hospital, and a midwife (not my usual midwife) came. We managed to persuade her to hand over to our midwife who was on duty that day from 8.30 am. I hadn't liked this unknown midwife, who told me I was 'distressed'.

"Although I hadn't been sure how my midwife would be, she gave me her entire attention and support. She and the student massaged my back in turns. I had a posterior labour. They made me feel cared for. Happy hours passed. I drank, walked about, ate honey and spent most of the late first stage sitting on a chair rocking or pushing against cushions on my high bed.

"I never considered pharmacological pain relief and coped with breathing. I also went into a trance-like state in between contractions and slept for a few minutes. The pain was strong but never overwhelming or frightening. The only painful times were when I started a contraction while being examined and when I tried being on all fours on the bed.

"When I was fully dilated the midwife came back into the room with the crib and baby clothes. This seemed unreal at the time – I didn't believe a baby would actually come out. There was no transition and no desire to push at all.

"It was decided that I was in the second stage, though, and they helped me to get on the bed in a semi-upright sitting position to push. As my body didn't want to do this, doubts about my ability to push a baby out started. The atmosphere became more tense and serious. My GP arrived, plus forceps bag. There was no descent, no progress. There was a general sinking feeling of hopes dashed. I struggled to hope something would change.

"An ambulance then arrived, and I calmly hopped into the back. I was fine and so was the baby, which at least meant there was no scary frantic rush. My husband followed in our car and so did my GP.

"When I arrived at hospital I was not allowed to walk, and put in a wheelchair. Staff I didn't know looked on with curiosity, but no one engaged with me. I was alone. My husband became increasingly scared and distant. I declined a monitor and was impressed with my assertion. A professor came in, came right up to me, and in a stage whisper told me mother had done well and now the professionals would take over (this was the gist of what he said, not his actual words). I remembered him from a conference where he had fallen asleep, and told him so loudly. I also insisted that if the baby didn't breathe in 5-10 minutes that they should not resuscitate. A drip was set up and a registrar said he would try ventouse (relief at not having forceps) and do a general anaesthetic Caesarean section if this didn't work (no time for an epidural).

"My contractions had weakened and I stopped doing anything with them. Luckily I was not in severe pain. The blackboard in the operating theatre had my name misspelt, which upset me. The ventouse was not painful, and my GP was in the operating theatre operating the footpump and complaining that it wasn't working. I had a large episiotomy and my baby was slowly drawn out like a cork. She was 8 lb 10 oz and alert (Apgar 9-10 at 1 minute, 10 out of 10 at 5 minutes). I was impressed by life and did feel it was a miracle. Later there was a gap because I had not seen her coming out or pushed her out myself.

"The hospital midwives thought I was having my second baby, and did not help with breastfeeding. However I did get visits from my midwife, GP, student; my main grouse was not having my husband beside me in the first euphoric hours. I also couldn't sleep as my bed was right next to the nursery. The routine of meals, etc., was comforting but also disorientating and I felt when coming home that I was returning from another planet.

"My second child was born at home on Christmas Eve and I greatly enjoyed the calm and family warmth of being able to sleep together with my husband, sisters and children."

Joanna O'Brien

"As soon as I found out I was pregnant I knew I wanted to have my baby at home. I felt strongly that I didn't want intervention and that we are designed to give birth naturally. My doctor was not welcoming and accommodating – she said 'of course it would be lovely if we could all give birth at home' but went on to describe a negative scenario and said I wouldn't want to be going over speed humps when I was in labour. I had been prepared for a fight and was quite defensive, but she didn't actually say no and wrote home birth on my referral letter.

"At my booking-in visit at 12 weeks the midwives were OK about it – even slightly excited – but they were too busy to discuss it then and said that they would come to my house to talk about it. This did not happen until I was about 6-7 months pregnant when she came with a whole list of potentially dangerous situations which she posed to see what my reaction was. I said that we would go in if there was a problem – that is what hospital is for. She also brought a letter saying that the hospital might not be able to provide a midwife to help me to have my baby at home – if there was a shortage of staff, I would have to come in to hospital – which gave me plenty of time to worry about it.

"There were no problems in pregnancy, I didn't get any negative feelings from the midwives, in fact they put me in touch with the home birth support group. However, I did not really see any one of them more than twice and I had to have shared care with my GP which seemed like a waste – I would have preferred to see the midwives all the time.

"My baby was due on New Year's Eve and I was concerned about getting a midwife over the holiday period – I couldn't get anyone to give me their mobile number.

"In fact I was 13 days over and booked for induction the following day when I went into labour. I had started feeling cramps, like period pains, very occasionally and gently in the evening. We went to bed at 10.30 pm, but I was up again at 11.30 pm as the pains were becoming stronger. I realised that this must be it and was too excited to sleep and wanted to be moving around. I wandered around the house, listened to some music, had a bath, ate some cereal and had a cup of tea. I rang the labour ward at about 4 am and they said I sounded far too happy to be in labour and to ring in the morning.

"The midwife came to see me in the morning at 8.30, then went on her rounds, telling me to ring if I needed her. By midday I was desperate to get in the pool that we had hired. I rang and she said she would come over so I waited. I knew if I got in too early there was a risk labour could slow down so I wanted the midwife to check me first and make sure I was over 5 cm. When she arrived, I was still only 3-4 cm dilated so I stayed out of the water. Contractions varied in strength, squatting made them stronger, but progress was slow. At 7.00 my midwife examined me – I was 7 cm but the baby's head was still high up and not pushing on my cervix. My waters went while I was being examined and we found old meconium in them. There wasn't a lot but it was enough to be sure.

"Our midwife was brilliant and discussed this with us in a very calm and measured way; she said that there was no need to panic but potentially it was a cause for concern and that we ought to think about going in. I asked her 'what would happen if I said no, no, no?' and she said 'it is entirely up to you'. I knew that she was pro-home birth so I didn't feel any pressure to go in. We discussed it for a good half-hour and decided that the best thing for the baby was to go in. It was my decision and felt like the right thing to do. I feel OK about it now too. She rang to let them know that we were coming.

"By the time we got there it was around 9.00. We'd had a delay leaving home as I hadn't fully packed my hospital bag thinking (hoping) I wouldn't need it. I took my shoes off at the delivery room door and my midwife said 'keep your shoes on for a minute and stand over there' – I saw what she meant – there was a small pool of blood on the floor, dried but still red. She cleared it up and then I was strapped to the monitors, unable to move around very much. My contractions were rubbish when I was standing up or leaning forward but splendid when I was lying on my back. They were still stopping and starting – I'd get a strong one and then a wussy one. Our midwife asked 'shall we try helping it along a bit?' I agreed as I just didn't seem to be making much headway and she put up a Syntocinon drip which helped a little. I was snoozing when the urge to push came on quite suddenly but there was a lip of cervix which held things up. I ended up lying on my back with one foot on my husband and one on the midwife with her actually holding the lip back as I pushed. She could see the head but it was still quite high up and it kept slipping back between contractions. There was no sign of fetal distress that

I was aware of (although from my notes it seems the baby's heart rate was not recovering as well as it should). Eventually she said 'I think we need some help – how do you feel about that?'. I said it was OK and a tiny little woman obstetrician came in and asked me if she could put in an epidural in case we had to go to theatre if the ventouse didn't work. I said no, we'd try the ventouse first and then decide what next if we needed to – I was quite clear-headed and together, I hadn't had any drugs. It turned out afterwards that she had thought we wouldn't be able to get her out – her head was still very high up.

"It took ages to get set up, they brought in the buffet trolley with the resucitation things on – lots of people in white coats came in, it was bizarre to be introduced to people and say 'hello, nice to meet you' when they were able to look right up you. I was in stirrups by then and had a local anaesthetic for the episiotomy, so I didn't really feel the catheter going in and then out. The first time they put the ventouse cap on and the head was nearly out, the cap came off. The second time they must have cut me and it came through. They said 'the head's out, the head's out' and the body slipped out with the next contraction. It was 4.05 am. They put her on my tummy and I touched her, she was warm and wet but didn't move. They cut the cord straightaway, then whipped her off and onto the trolley. She did not breath for a minute or so, her Apgar was low and her hands and feet were quite blue. They gave her some oxygen and when she was crying she was put back. It wasn't long. The obstetrician got on with the repair and the lights were so bright. She was given to me wrapped – I unwrapped her and held her against my skin and tried to shield her eyes from such a rude awakening. She had been born very suddenly after 27 hours of labour. After a while she stopped crying and started calmly considering me with one open eye, she was alert and taking it all in, she seemed to be watching my face intently.

"My blood pressure was very low and I lost a lot of blood so I had to wait in the delivery room for it to settle. I had a shower while my husband helped the student midwife give her a bath. I felt quite light-headed then and wanted to sit on one of the benches but I kept thinking that I couldn't as I had an open wound and did not want to expose it to all those germs.

"Two nurses came and took me up to the ward at about 6.30

am. I went in a wheelchair holding my baby while they carried my bag. They left me sitting on the edge of a bed and said they would be back to help me into bed. It seems that they forgot – I was left sitting there watching it grow light outside and looking at my beautiful baby. I wanted to get into bed but didn't know how to move holding a baby and I was just exhausted, I could hardly move my legs from tiredness. I was eventually rescued by the woman who came round with the tea. We had to stay in overnight because of the meconium although there wasn't much of it in the water. They wanted to monitor my baby's chest.

"I'm fairly philosophical about it having been the right place to have had her. I'm still not clear what was causing the problem, it really seemed like she just didn't want to come out. I had quite severe symphysis pubis pain for several months afterwards, as though it had overstretched. I have taken my daughter to a cranial osteopath because of the ventouse and also because if my pubic bone was this sore, her head must have suffered too. I asked my midwife if I would have done better on my hands and knees, and she said it would've been better for my pelvis but wouldn't have helped the contractions since they only happened effectively on my back.

"I've examined my feelings closely and it felt like the right thing to do. Although it was a long way from how I planned it I don't feel traumatised, I think because I was making the decisions along the way and had a very supportive midwife. I was disappointed not to use the pool though. Next time it will be different."

Jo

"My daughter, Lizmiah, was a home water birth. I was not really very good around the medical profession – least of all, hospitals – and preferred to take charge of my own health. So with both a birthing and a water birth course at the Active Birth Centre, and homeopathic remedies supplied by my homeopath, I decided to plump for a birth at home.

"It was really lovely not having to worry about when to go in, or when not to go in, to hospital. I must have had quite strong contractions for at least a week preceding the actual birth but, of course, I did not actually have to think about whether or not 'this was it' but could wait and see how things panned out, trusting that I would know when it really was full on. Boy did I know! When labour started in earnest I went straight into major contractions, every five minutes – but I wouldn't let my husband call the midwife until they had done this for at least one hour (which is what we had been told to wait for!). By the time she arrived, I was already five centimetres dilated and could get straight into the pool.

"The pool was WONDERFUL – so warm and calming and 'holding'. The only down-side to it, in hindsight, was that I found myself staying in the same position (on my knees with my legs spayed out at the hips) for nearly the entire eleven hour birth and I wonder if that was to keep my body submerged as much as possible for maximum pain relief. On the other hand, it could be that this was simply my way of dealing with what was initially a transverse birthing position.

"Lizmiah's birth was not an easy one and I genuinely feel that if she had been a hospital birth she would have ended up as a Caesarean. She started out in a transverse position, which was really painful, and remained that way for quite a long time. I don't know at what point she eventually turned since I thought she had actually been born posterior but, in a debrief years later with the midwife in charge, I found out that she had not. Then, just when I thought things were going really well and she would be born within the hour, it turned out that I had an anterior lip (probably because of her positioning) and that all my pushing and pain were not actually going anywhere. I used homeopathy and we kept going for another hour but to no avail and the midwife decided at that point, having consulted with me and asked my permission, to push the lip back manually. She apologised a lot about how painful this procedure was but, I have to admit, I did not actually feel a thing compared to the transverse labour I was already experiencing!

"The second stage of labour began and took about two hours or so, Lizmiah seeming to get stuck in the lower birth canal for about an hour until the midwife helped me find another way of pushing (just when I was really feeling that it would never end and wondering how much longer I could go on). I was told later in my debrief that this is quite a long time for a second stage – they normally like it to be no longer than an hour and a half –

but that the midwife stuck by me because although things were moving very slowly they were always moving nonetheless. That and the fact that my daughter's amazing little heart beat was so strong and steady and never changed from the beginning to the end of labour. This, however, is the point at which I really feel a home birth was on my side. I do not think that they would have been prepared to wait that long had I been in a hospital room. I think the urge to 'hurry me on' or to use readily-available intervention would have been irresistible. As it was, the midwife sat quietly and attentively on the sidelines leaving me in charge of my birth and consulting me on all decisions. I had a huge sac of waters, for instance, which did not break until probably about a third of the way through the second stage. The midwife had offered earlier to break them for me but, when asked, had said that there was no particular reason why this would help and so I had decided to leave them intact, reasoning that, although it was painful, if they had not yet broken naturally, maybe nature had her reasons. I later was told in the debrief that, in a transverse or posterior birth such as Lizmiah's, it is good when the waters remain intact for as long as possible since they can exert an even pressure on the cervix, something the head is unable to do when in the wrong position, and thus avert an anterior lip. Didn't work in my case but was at least worth a try!

"The other great thing about having a home birth was how much it facilitated my feeling of being in control and able to make my own decisions. It felt very much as if the midwives had entered my space – they were my guests and were there to aid me. It was primarily my birthing experience in my home – all my surroundings were familiar and comforting, I knew where everything was, I chose to use homeopathy and that was OK and natural because it was a part of what always went on in this household. Birthing simply felt like an extension of my usual lifestyle as it were; something very extraordinary happening in a very ordinary way. Therefore, when two or three doctors arrived on my doorstep early into the labour and wanted to sit in on the proceedings since they had never been party to a home water birth before, I was able to ask them to leave after I discovered it was significantly affecting my ability to birth. Likewise I was able to ask the poor student midwife to sit in my kitchen whilst I gave birth in the lounge, having previously discovered I was no good at 'performing'. I certainly would not have felt anywhere near as comfortable with these requests, probably unable to make them, had I been in their territory and not my own.

"When Lizmiah was finally born she did not manage to take on breathing for any length of time. The midwife reports that she would breathe briefly and turn pink and healthy and then stop and turn pale and floppy. The fact that in order to have a home birth you must have at least one senior and one or two other midwives present stood us in good stead here. I had three midwives present at this point (two of them senior) – and the student in the kitchen! The leading midwife was very calm and clear and also very quick and thorough. She tried various natural techniques to get my baby breathing fully – putting her at the breast, rubbing her vigorously with a towel, slapping her gently – and for this I am very grateful. Had I been in a hospital I wonder whether, for a start, I would have had such an experienced midwife already with me (let alone so many of them) but I also wonder whether there would not have been the temptation to rush straight to the doctors and the technology. As it was, when Lizmiah did not respond to any of these un-invasive methods two of the midwives used an oxygen mask and pumped air into her until an ambulance came for her and she was transferred to hospital with my husband accompanying her. I followed on later in a separate ambulance with the second senior midwife (who was supposed to deliver my placenta at home first – but that is another story for another time!).

"Lizmiah spent six days in hospital with myself, four of them in intensive care. When she arrived they were not sure if they had the specialist care for her but within one hour she had torn out her tubes and continued to go from strength to strength. No one knows to this day why she did not breathe, although various tests were done. I do not feel that the home birth was detrimental to her in any way. She received excellent care the whole time and medical treatment was available to her quickly when she needed it. And yet we both still got to have a good birthing experience. We were laughing at her strong and unchanging heartbeat by the end of the birth – it did not change even when she was not breathing.

"I certainly have no regrets. I went on to have my second child at home too (no complications at all – a three minute second stage in comparison!). This time it was a delight to experience the sheer magic and bliss of home aftercare where we all sat around having a cup of tea whilst I breastfed him and the midwife poured us a bath before putting me to bed with my newborn son whilst she cleaned up my lounge! Absolutely magical!"

Sam Cairns

12   problems after birth

'FLAT' BABY

Very occasionally a baby is born 'flat' or limp and showing no inclination to breathe, even though there has been no indication of
fetal distress during labour. It is a condition that is often feared by
those opposed to home birth and, although it is very unlikely, it is
a possibility that has to be considered.

Once delivered, a baby may quite normally not breathe for at
least 30 seconds. This can seem like a lifetime to its parents but has
no ill effect on the baby. In fact babies can survive far longer than
adults without oxygen; it takes 12 minutes before its lack starts to
cause brain damage.

If the baby has not started to breathe within one minute the
midwife will take steps to help it. After sucking out any mucus from
the baby's mouth or throat she will put a small mask over its face
and puff oxygen over it. It is important that the cord is not cut at
this point as it continues to provide the baby with oxygen as long
as it is still pulsating. The baby should also be kept warm.

If the baby is still not breathing the midwife will put a tight-fit-
ting mask over its mouth and nose and force oxygen into its lungs
by means of an Ambubag. An airway helps to ensure that it goes
into the lungs and not the stomach. In most cases these measures
will be effective, so that the baby is breathing within two or three
minutes.

If the baby still does not breathe, someone should call an ambulance. Anyone can do this – the medical attendants will be engaged
in resuscitating the baby. The midwives or doctor present will also
try mouth to mouth resuscitation by putting their mouth over the
baby's mouth and nose and puffing air in gently. If the heartbeat
drops below 60 beats per minute they will also start giving the
baby heart massage. When the paramedics arrive they will administer

oxygen by passing an endotracheal tube into the baby's lungs and pumping oxygen directly into them. It must be done by someone experienced in the technique of intubation as there is a risk of misplacing the tube so that it is either ineffective or damaging. Once this is set up it will be connected to the ventilator in the incubator and the baby will be transferred to hospital.

Intubation is a technique not usually immediately available at a home delivery and you must consider how you might feel if your baby should ultimately need this kind of resuscitation. There is a controversial view among some midwives that strong babies will always make it and that those which require this type of care may be brain damaged. There is no firm evidence to support this view, but you may have definite ideas about whether you would prefer your child to survive at any price or whether you would rather it did not live than go through life disabled.

How you can help your baby

If possible hold the baby while it is being helped to breathe. Stroke it and tell it why you want it here. Flick the soles of its feet with your fingers. You can put Bach's rescue remedy into the baby's mouth and on the pulse points at wrist and temples. Take some yourselves.

If your baby is not breathing and there is no one there to help you, you can put your own mouth over its mouth and nose and puff small but frequent breaths of air in.

If its heart is not beating, put your hand under its back and press down on its sternum with your thumb with as much pressure as would dent raw pastry. Repeat this as often and as quickly as you can.

POSTPARTUM HAEMORRHAGE

This is the other emergency which causes anxiety about home birth. It is less likely to occur at home than in hospital (0.3 per cent at home and 1.1 per cent in hospital in a Dutch study). Recent NICE analysis is more ambivalent but it does not feature in every study they analysed. It is more common following induction and acceleration of labour. It is frightening when it does occur, not least because of the rate at which blood can be lost. Primary postpartum haemorrhage is classified as a blood loss exceeding 500 ml, the amount which is regarded as normal in a healthy mother. It can occur for several reasons, all of which can be treated at home, although in some circumstances it may mean that you need to be transferred to hospital thereafter. They include the following.

Bad tear or episiotomy

This will require clamping of the bleeding points with the artery forceps, and subsequent suturing. Very severe tears may require suturing in hospital, but most can be repaired at home. Some, but not all, midwives have been trained to suture. If your midwife cannot do it she is able to call a doctor who will.

Vulval varicosity

Varicose veins in the vulva can bleed badly if they are damaged at birth. The bleeding can be staunched by holding a sanitary pad firmly against the area of rupture until it can be repaired.

Cervical tears

If your uterus is contracted and the cause of bleeding is not directly visible, an ambulance will be called. If bleeding is coming from a laceration of your cervix, you will be given an intravenous transfusion of fluids and transferred to hospital for a surgical repair.

Atonic uterus

This is where the uterus fails to contract after the delivery of the baby so that the raw area left by the detached placenta remains large and free to bleed. Normally it contracts down, constricting the blood vessels so that the bleeding stops.

The uterus is likely to contract once the placenta has been delivered if you have had a normal first, second and third stage, if you are not inhibited by those around you, and if all is well with the baby. Atonic uterus is more common when labour is induced or accelerated.

It is to prevent postpartum haemorrhage that Syntometrine is given routinely. This is a combination of synthetic oxytocin and ergometrine that is usually given by injection into the mother's thigh as the baby's shoulders are delivered. It has the effect of contracting the uterus down hard within seven minutes. This reduces the incidence of bleeding, but increases the incidence of retained placentas.

This is because unless the placenta is delivered before the uterus contracts, it may be trapped within it, which may mean that it has to be pulled out. Moreover the cord has to be cut immediately if the contracting uterus is not to pump extra, unnecessary blood into the baby.

For these reasons women giving birth at home often choose to do without Syntometrine, feeling that if they have managed up until then without aid, their bodies are likely to complete the third stage unaided as well, and NICE guidelines support a physiological third stage in low-risk women. In less natural circumstances you might want to accept Syntometrine. If you do not and then do start to bleed from the uterus you will be given ergometrine into a vein. This will act to contract the uterus down in 45 seconds. In the unlikely event of this failing to stop the bleeding, the midwife would stimulate a contraction by rubbing your abdomen over the uterus, insert a urinary catheter and administer pressure by squeezing your uterus bimanually with one hand in your vagina. In the meantime the ambulance will have been called and would arrive bringing equipment for intravenous infusion, and you would be transferred to hospital.

How you can help yourself

Bleeding is thought to be unlikely to occur if you take the homeopathic remedies Arnica and Kali Phos at the birth. Make sure that you urinate hourly in labour so that the bladder is empty when you give birth. If bleeding occurs, get someone to put a bit of the placenta, if delivered, into your mouth and pinch your ankle hard at the point between your ankle bones. Maintain the pressure until the bleeding stops. Put your baby to your breast. Sip half a cup of warm water to which has been added a teaspoon of cayenne pepper.

A serious tear or episiotomy is less likely if you have massaged your perineum daily from around 30 weeks of pregnancy. It can also help to soften previous episiotomy scars. Try the massage after a warm bath. Lubricate your fingers with an oil such as comfrey, almond, olive or vitamin E, or an ointment like calendula or comfrey. Then very gently insert two fingers into your vagina and gradually separate them so that the skin of the vagina becomes stretched, a bit like pulling at the corners of your mouth. With practice you will be able to expand your vagina more and more. Next hook your thumb into your vagina and pull the perineum outward, using oil to massage the skin in a U-shape, concentrating on any previous scar or area of tenderness.

WOMEN'S STORIES

"I chose to have my second baby at home because I had had a domino delivery for my first and, although I was really pleased with it, I felt I hadn't needed to go in. I don't like hospitals and only five minutes after Jennifer was born I thought that I would have the next one at home. I didn't want any intervention which I had avoided with the first birth, largely because she was born at the crack of dawn on a Sunday morning before a bank holiday.

"Before I went into labour I had a false start on Tuesday night, which had stopped by the morning. I spoke to the midwife, who advised me to keep my clinic appointment the following afternoon, which was the day the baby was due. She then rang back and said she would visit me later that afternoon instead. I went to my antenatal class the next morning where everyone was very excited as they thought I was going to have it there. I felt I didn't know what was going to happen but I went home and sat around in the afternoon. By mid-afternoon the contractions had started again but they weren't bad – just like strong period pains. The midwife eventually came at 6.30, but the contractions weren't anything to worry about, and she went home.

"I wandered round tidying up, watched Coronation Street and put Jennifer to bed. We got the bedroom ready and then I had a bath. I timed the contractions, which I hadn't bothered to do before, and found they were coming every five minutes and lasting for about one minute. At 9.30 I got out of the bath and standing up seemed to start things moving. I got dressed in loose clothing and at 10.00 we called the midwife, who arrived with a student. Half an hour later one of the other midwives arrived too. At this point I wanted to lean over my husband in the bedroom, but the midwife felt I was too curved and suggested squatting would speed things up. The bed was the wrong height and so we moved into the bathroom. We found a position where Paul sat on the bath and I squatted with my elbows on his knees. I needed the window open; it had been stifling in the bedroom and I think I really wanted to give birth outside.

"I used that position in the bathroom for each contraction for about an hour while the midwives were downstairs having quite a party. I could hear them laughing and I had told them where the chocolate biscuits were. After a while they sat on the landing and left us to it, checking every 15 minutes or so. They were waiting for the grunting sounds to get worse before they came in. I didn't feel an urge to push, but I was sick twice before I started to push and they said that was a good sign, that the baby would soon be there. I got a big cuddle from them which was really nice. It did hurt more than I remembered with Jennifer and I felt very impatient, although I didn't say anything. Eventually I said 'I need help'. I remember thinking I just wanted someone to put a hand in and pull her out, it seemed so obvious, but of course it wasn't to be.

"In fact it was a very straightforward delivery, I was almost standing up, crouched over with Paul supporting me. She was born in the bedroom with the television on showing *Match of the Day*. We had got the soft lights and music all ready but we didn't get round to it. We had had them with Jennifer, but it all seemed so matter of fact this time. The dog came up to see what was happening and then the cat; the midwife had to put them out in the end and the dog stood outside the house barking.

"The baby was placed on to my lap as I sat on the end of the bed. I waited for the placenta to be delivered and Roisin gasped intermittently and did not breathe properly. I became aware that the midwives were getting worried, but I felt instinctively that everything would be all right. I was concerned with delivering the placenta, which came away later, naturally but painfully, into Jennifer's potty as the bucket was in the other room.

"I heard the midwife say 'Shall we call the flying squad' and I was aware of one midwife coming in and out of the bedroom, using the oxygen, flicking Roisin's feet, and another saying 'Aren't they here yet?' I didn't get any feeling that there was any real need for concern as she was still on my lap and the cord was still pulsing. I think Paul was more worried than I was. In fact it was 13 minutes before Roisin was breathing properly. At this point (20 minutes after the initial call) they asked me if I wanted to go in and I said I certainly did not, so they rang to cancel the flying squad. The really worrying thing was that the squad had not even left the hospital, because they had not been able to get an ambulance. I later heard the registrar had said that 'by now the baby is either all right or it's dead'.

"After this we put a hat on the baby and went to bed."

Lucy McAteer

"It was snowing on the afternoon of 27 April, which in retrospect seemed to be auspicious. We were awaiting the birth of our third child. I had been booked for home birth in all my pregnancies, but my first baby had been breech at 36 weeks and so had been delivered in hospital. My second child had been born at home normally without any problems.

"William was nine days overdue, as the others had been, and his head was not engaged, when shortly before three in the afternoon the head engaged suddenly as I rushed to help Thomas who had poured a bottle of white spirit over his head. By about four, while at a children's party, I was aware my waters were going, so I sat down for a bit. Contractions started, and seemed to be quite strong. We got home at six and by then I had a lot of low abdominal pain. We phoned the midwife at 6.15 and she arrived at about 7.00. She gave me an internal examination and said I wasn't at all dilated. However, contractions were coming thick and fast and so she decided to stay.

"We rang a friend who was going to be with us for the birth and she arrived bringing her transcutaneous nerve stimulator. I had a long bath while the children were put to bed. At about 9.00 I felt that although the bath was helping with the pain, I had better get out in order to put on the TENS, which did definitely work. At 8.55 I was examined again and found to be 3 cm. The contractions were by then every three minutes and growing increasingly strong. I was walking about, stopping still for each one.

"At 9.30 the back-up midwife arrived, bringing her student with her. By 10.25 I had the urge to push and positioned myself half-sitting, half squatting, on the end of our bed. Christopher was behind me, our original midwife had one leg, my friend the other, the student was ready to deliver the baby and the second midwife was sitting in a chair, watching. The baby's heartbeat had been checked at regular intervals and all seemed well. Second stage was not particularly long and at 10.43 William was born, weighing 9 lb 3 oz.

"He was blue and did not breathe. At first this did not seem important but as time went by there was increasing concern. He was given oxygen from a cylinder and mouth to mouth resuscitation was applied. The room was not warm enough, as he arrived before the temperature had been raised for the birth, and I could not see what was happening as he was being resuscitated on the window seat with the midwife between him and me. I was so exhausted that I could not feel anything more than mild concern, although I could see that Christopher was worried. I felt that there were so many people there that I couldn't contribute anything. By 10.55 William was breathing by himself, roughly but constantly. His heartbeat had remained strong throughout. He was very cold.

"During this time the flying squad had been called from the hospital about 3 miles away and at 11.10 two ambulances arrived, one containing the paediatric registrar and a hospital midwife. After we were both examined and there was some discussion, William and I were taken to hospital. Christopher had to follow by car.

"William went to special care, accompanied by Christopher. This was principally to warm him rather than because he had any further problem with his breathing. We were told the first 24 hours would be critical.

"I was stitched and bathed and taken to bed. I went to see William at five the next morning. We stayed in for 36 hours.

"William is now two and developmentally fine. I feel that the way he arrived was just one of those things that happened; in hospital he would only have been ventilated earlier, which wasn't necessary as he breathed in his own time. At the time I did not worry about it, although subsequently I have thought about what might have happened. The experience would not deter me from another home birth were I to have another baby."

Catherine Gash
(And indeed three and a half years later Catherine gave birth to Rosamund, entirely without problems, at home. See Eleanor's story on page 141).

"I did not decide to have a home delivery until late in my pregnancy, for a number of reasons. During my career as a midwife and health visitor I had never been involved in a home delivery – I simply did not consider it as an option. We were in the process of moving house and I could not be sure where I would be for the baby's birth. I must admit that I felt the need to conform, not to be different or difficult.

"My attitude changed, I believe, due to the tour of the hospital (where I had worked as a midwife) and the NCT antenatal classes I attended. I had also given up work, so had more time to reflect on my pregnancy and the fast approaching birth. The NCT classes gave me the confidence to make the decision to have my baby in comfortable, familiar surroundings. Although I had worked at the hospital, seeing the labour ward as a pregnant woman made me feel frightened and uneasy. It seemed so clinical, with equipment available for every kind of intervention possible; I had already decided I wanted minimum intervention.

"I informed my GP, the community midwives and the hospital of my decision to have my baby at home. My GP felt very strongly that I should be delivered in hospital but finally agreed to attend the birth. The manager of the community midwives visited me and did her utmost to change my mind, to no avail. The hospital consultant advised me against home delivery, but did agree that I was a good candidate, as my pregnancy had progressed so well to date. There were times when I almost relented, the worst accusation being that my baby's well-being would be threatened by a home delivery. However by now I was determined to have a home delivery, provided all continued to progress normally.

"I was in early labour when I first met the midwife who was to deliver my baby; she was very kind and I had every confidence in her. We agreed that I should sleep and contact her when the contractions became stronger and more regular. Gary (my husband), on hearing that I was not in too much pain, decided to work late. It was on his return (and after a short lecture about husbands supporting their wives in labour), that my contractions became regular and much more painful. I discovered that I wanted to labour alone, so as it was 11 pm Gary went to bed and I retired to our spare room with a hot water bottle. I found that squatting on the floor during contractions helped to ease the pain and I managed to doze in between. Finally, I decided that I would try the TENS machine which I had hired. Gary was by now awake, so he prepared the room and tried to decipher the TENS machine instructions.

"Eventually, with the machine set up and working, my waters broke and I decided it was time to call the midwife. Before she arrived I had the urge to push, but managed to control it until she confirmed that I was fully dilated. My GP arrived soon afterwards, and everyone (except me) sat down and had a nice cup of tea. The midwife was wonderful – on a request for instructions she advised me to follow my instincts. I spent the second stage of labour on all fours, pushing when and for as long as I felt necessary. My daughter was born at 5 am, a normal delivery of a beautiful baby. I had almost forgotten about the third stage of labour, a mere formality, surely. I wanted a cup of tea.

"However, despite our efforts, I had a retained placenta and the flying squad were called. Gary, our baby and myself were then taken to hospital in an ambulance, having had a drip set up and blood taken for cross matching should I need a transfusion. My placenta was manually removed under a general anaesthetic, and I was in hospital for 24 hours.

"I felt that a retained placenta and all the consequences were simply bad luck. I did feel sorry not to spend those first few hours at home, but I had achieved my main objective – I had delivered a beautiful baby following a normal delivery at home."

Paula Ayres
(Since then Paula has had another baby at home – a boy, born without any complications and without syntometrine.)

Transfer

As these stories show – the way women feel about transfer depends on how necessary it seemed to be. Hospital interventions can be genuinely lifesaving, and many women and babies have died in childbirth who could have been saved with modern obstetrical techniques. Women who are convinced that they needed help are usually disappointed but thankful. Women who have planned and looked forward to home birth only to have to transfer on questionable grounds can, understandably, feel quite bitter.

If you do have to transfer, don't give up on all your ambitions. There is no need to conform to hospital routine – try and make the space as personal and private as possible. Ask your midwife to help people stay out unless you need immediate medical help. Ask for the lights to be lowered and for there to be no talking during contractions. You can go home as soon as you have had the baby if there are no contraindications. If you have to stay in, make sure that you are well-supplied with water and fresh food including protein, fruit and vegetables.

It will be important to debrief and find out what went right and what went wrong. If this opportunity is not offered to you, ask to see the midwife with whom you transferred so that you can go through it with her in detail.

Don't feel that you can't go back to your home birth support group, who should be extra supportive, and don't feel a failure. Hindsight is a wonderful thing and the decisions you make at the time will be made without its benefit.

"My third child arrived in two hours and I planned a home water birth for my fourth – the others having been born at home in England, America and Australia.

"I had a show the Thursday before and then niggles and contractions over the next few days but nothing really getting established. Monday afternoon, around 4 pm the contractions became more regular (5 mins) and stronger. I called my husband home from work and began to prepare for labour – convinced that this was it. Three hours on, there was no change but we felt we should let the hospital know as they had warned us that there might be a shortage of midwives. Sure enough when I phoned they told me that there would be no one available until

8 am the next day. I tried calling some of the community mid-wives on their mobiles but they were unable to come too. At this point I became quite tearful. My husband went into assertive mode and called the hospital back insisting that they send someone out and that there was no way we were coming in.

"It worked. And a young midwife came out to assess me. I knew I wasn't in established labour and we had tried to explain this to the hospital but I think they were making a point and sent her anyway. When she arrived my contractions all but disappeared. She also offered me a sweep which I refused. As she was leaving Berny, who made the Homebirth Diaries and was making a new programme about home birth, arrived. She asked the midwife if she would mind being filmed – the midwife was not sure and left to go back to the hospital.

"As soon as she had gone my contractions picked up again and I went to my room to labour privately. After an hour the contractions were strong and coming every 2-3 mins so we phoned the hospital again. Again they said there was no one available, again my husband had to argue with them and they sent 2 midwives. The hospital also made it clear that they did not want their midwives filmed even though Berny had previously cleared it with the head of midwifery and the PR department.

"When the midwives arrived labour continued with me using my ball and TENS. I was 4 cm dilated increasing to 5 on a contraction. I was surprised that this labour was taking so long – it had been 8 hours now – the same length as my first. After a while I got in the pool. This seemed to speed things along a bit and I felt I was in transition although it did not seem that intense. I also got an urge to push but again it was not that strong so I held back remindful of my second labour when I had an anterior lip. I mentioned this to the midwives but they seemed unconcerned and just told me to listen to my body. After a time of pushing with contractions getting stronger and longer there was still no baby. This again was concerning to me as during my last labour I hardly needed to push at all, she just slipped out.

"After the next contraction the midwife listened to the baby's heartbeat and it was dangerously low. She tried to feel the baby's head on the next contraction but felt a lip [incomplete dilation where a small area of cervix holds the baby back] instead. I KNEW IT! I was so disappointed and tired I just kind of gave up and started to cry. I asked the midwife if she could push it back and got out the pool and lay on the couch. The contractions were agony and I chugged on the gas and air which the midwives encouraged. Through my druggy haze (I couldn't see and hardly hear because I had so much) I heard the words ambulance and c-section mentioned. It transpired that the baby was showing concerning signs of distress and that the ambulance was on its way. If the baby didn't arrive before I got to the hospital then I would have an emergency Caesarean section.

"The midwife pushed the lip back and Stella shot out like a torpedo in a Niagara falls of amniotic fluid (yes, the sofa will never be the same again). On my notes it reads 2nd stage 2 mins. The cord was cut immediately and Stella was taken away as she wasn't breathing and needed to be given oxygen and resuscitated. I was left on the couch with Berny (who had now taken on the role of doula rather than camerawoman) reassuring me. I was really scared – I hadn't even seen my baby before she was taken and no one was telling me what was going on. It was only when the ambulance men walked in to my living-room that I got to see her. I was given Syntometrine also at this point so I could go in the ambulance with her. By the time we left the house she was looking good – had a good colour and was breathing normally.

"On arrival she was checked over by a paediatrician and everything looked good. Finally, an hour after her birth I could hold her. She fed immediately and I was so relieved, disappointed and happy about the birth, the labour, the hospital, everything, I was quite overwhelmed. However, the hospital wanted to keep her in for observation so we were transferred to a postnatal ward. My heart goes out to all women who have had to endure postnatal wards at this point – I won't go into moany details but by 7 am I was in tears and threatening to get the bus home. Luckily my husband went into assertive role again and made sure the doctor saw us first and by lunchtime we were home.

"I am so happy that everything was ok in the end but I can't help feeling disappointed that the birth was so dramatic and completely different to what I wanted. It was stressful from the start with the lack of midwives and the tension between the hospital and us demanding to be seen and also their problems with Berny. I also feel the midwives should have picked up on the lip sooner as I did tell them of my fears (and listened to my body). Stella is doing really well and seems none the worse for her dramatic first hour in this world. I have also had time to process what happened and asked questions. It appears that the midwife who delivered her was a hospital midwife rather than a community midwife and so was unused to home birth. Basically she panicked when Stella shot out and cut the cord too early so depriving Stella of her much needed oxygen. The midwife did exactly what she would do in hospital circumstances when you buzz for a paediatrician. As there obviously wasn't one she completely overreacted and sent us all off to hospital even though Stella was perfectly okay by the time we left the house.

"I still feel robbed of my home birth experience and of those precious first moments with my baby, all because of a hospital's lack of resources and mismanagement, but I'm sure these feelings will pass and I will put my anger to a more constructive use. However there is no damage done to Stella's and my relationship and we're both thriving. The treatment in the PN ward was the yucky, green icing on the cake.

"However, on a positive note I have learnt huge amounts going through this experience which I can bring to my doulaing and of course I have the most gorgeous, healthy little girl at the end of it."

Debra Flynn

"When we found out that Maria and I were expecting a baby, I just assumed that the hospital was the place to have it. After all there were lots of people and machines to cover all eventualities. So when she said that she wanted to have the baby at home, it came as a shock to me. I pretended to be open to the idea, knowing full well that she'd come to her senses sooner or later, once all the facts and statistics were in. What could be safer than a hospital?

"But as we did our research – partly based on an earlier, well-thumbed edition of this book – I couldn't really come up with any good arguments to support the idea of going to hospital like everyone else. And everyone seemed to want to tell me a horror story about home birth, but couldn't think of any. But there were so few women giving birth at home anyway, so even positive stories were hard to come by. So a home birth was it for us – not too difficult to obtain – but deep in my heart I was still longing for the 'safety' of a hospital.

"When labour started, I of course was the one who wanted to have the midwife there as soon as possible. Although I had settled for a home birth, the prospect of a birth at home without at least one midwife was very scary. But as the contractions were irregular, it was too early for her to come. When the contractions became more regular, I got my way and the midwife was called. She promptly arrived. We had met her a few times before, and were so happy that she was doing home births, that we failed to notice that she was hardly a home birth enthusiast. But here we were, it was all set to go, but the initial excitement gave way to a waiting game...

"Labour lasted for many hours and Maria made little progress. I became very aware that we kept a stranger waiting, who surely had better things to do, and who was getting tired, and seemed bored with the books she had brought. It seemed quite clear that if our midwife had to go, there would be no ready replacement for her. So when after 20 hours of labour, the midwife said it was best to go to hospital to put Maria on a drip, we were disappointed, but we were all so exhausted that it seemed like the most sensible option.

"The hospital was bright and busy and full of all the doctors, midwifes and nurses I could have wished for. I was now playing the role of the traditional father, a mediator between hospital staff and wife, with no responsibility but to keep by Maria's side and step away when others needed access to her.

"Our home birth midwife, exhausted, left, and another one we had never met before took her place. As Maria needed a drip to speed up dilation, our unborn baby was hooked up to a heartbeat monitor. Finally I thought, no more risks! We could even hear the baby's heartbeat! Then it abruptly stopped, but no one seemed to pay any attention. Almost embarrassed, I asked why the heartbeat had stopped. The nurse made some adjustment, and the healthy, fast heartbeat of our son once again be heard, only to stop again after a short while. After the third or fourth time, I finally realised that he wasn't about to die, and stopped paying attention.

"Did we want an epidural? Maria was in quite a bit of pain by now, and anyway a natural birth was out of the window, so we agreed. An anaesthetist came, performed the epidural, which took ages to work and then only worked partly, only adding to her discomfort.

"When still not much happened after a couple of hours, we got introduced to yet another midwife, who showed her disappointment at the slow progress. While slow progress at home had been difficult with one midwife waiting, slow progress at hospital seemed to attract even more disapproval, by the scores of very busy people. In the meantime, other, more 'capable' women around us seemed to be delivering babies much faster than we could manage. What was wrong with us? And in the meantime the room seemed to be getting brighter and busier, and I didn't any longer feel in safe hands. I longed to be back home, longed for a second chance to do it all differently. For the first time I began to wonder if all these health professionals really knew what they were doing, and whether I as a husband had not failed bringing my wife into this hell of a hospital birth.

"Then, just as this nightmare seemed to not want to end, a wonderful thing happened: midwife number four appeared, introduced herself kindly, closed the door, took one look at the room, and switched off the ceiling light. Suddenly the atmosphere changed – it was relaxing, quiet and the pressure seemed to be off. We were alone with her and our unborn baby. The best way to describe the room was that it was almost like being at home. From being exhausted and out of control, within a few minutes I became insanely happy: I was about to become a father. Maria also became more relaxed, she soon was fully dilated and, helped by an angel of a midwife, who seemed to say the right things at the right time, Maria seemingly effortlessly gave birth to our son Misha a few minutes before midnight, over 27 hours after labour started.

"We went home as quickly as we were allowed, trying to make up for the lost home birth as quickly as possible. As Misha, our son, took a first look at his home, I finally understood that hospital was a place for sick people, not a place to give birth. And I knew what I wanted for the next birth: of course it had to be at home and, even more importantly, it had to be a midwife we would feel comfortable to keep waiting, and who would agree that the best place to give birth was home.

"For the next pregnancy, three years later, we signed up with a group of midwives who specialised in home births (which coincidentally, but not entirely surprisingly included the midwife who had delivered Misha!). I took an active part in organising everything, much more than I had for the first planned home birth, determined that everything would go right. We hired a birthing pool from a place in the middle of nowhere, where house numbers were apparently not required but would have been very useful. The pool was ready weeks early and served as a swimming pool for Misha and us over the weeks of waiting, adding to the sense of excitement. There was no sense of the dread on my part which had accompanied the uncertainty of the first birth.

"I still remember Misha's amazed expression when he woke up in the morning and had his first look at Hannah who had been born at dawn. A perfect water birth, relaxed and stress free. The labour had been 20 hours shorter than with Misha. And then, around the same time 18 months later, Misha and Hannah crept down the stairs to take a first look at their sister Jodie, also born in a pool. I was a home birth convert – only problem being is that selling your house where your children were born would probably be just a little more heartbreaking. But we'll hang on to it just a little while longer."

Martin Wagner

13   death at birth

On rare occasions – statistically more rarely than in hospital – a baby delivered at home dies, either before it is born or shortly afterwards. This is always a tragedy and there really is no consolation. However there are aspects of stillbirth or neonatal death at home from which bereaved families draw some comfort. (If you feel that your baby would not have died if you had been in hospital then the following considerations will be of no help at all.)

If his or her death seems to be inevitable or unpreventable, you may prefer that your baby is born at home. The baby will then be born into his or her home, with the benefits that labour at home brings; you will be freer than in hospital to express your grief; and you will be in your own surroundings with the rest of your family around you if you wish. You will not be among other women who have given birth to healthy babies. Once the baby is born you can spend as long as you like with him or her – the decision about when the baby leaves the house is up to you, and you can feel that he or she has been home, even though they may not have been aware of it. If you feel that home is the right place to be born, you may also feel it is the right place to die.

If your baby is born alive at home but is clearly not going to live and is unable to benefit from hospital treatment, then you may prefer that his or her short life is spent in your home where you can make the most of the time that you have together. You may prefer that the baby dies there in your arms rather than in a hospital side-room, where you are dependent on the skill of the staff to handle the situation with tact and sympathy.

There are, of course, many staff in hospital with just such skills, but even then death, as so often with birth, may be sanitised and regulated so that a baby can seem to belong more to the hospital than to you, and the opportunity to spend time with your dead child can be limited to what other people feel you can take. Birth and death have today been removed from everyday life so that most people have seen neither – a situation that is far removed from that of people in the past. If your baby is born dead or dies at home, then you can spend as much time as you want looking at it, touching it, holding it, cuddling it and finally saying goodbye to it. You can take photos as you wish and build up some memory of your baby, so that when he or she is no longer there you are not grieving in a vacuum.

Clearly, facing these issues demands a strength and courage that you may feel you do not have. After all, many women having still-born babies in hospital feel that they cannot bear to look at their child, although they may subsequently regret it. However, as things stand at the moment, the sort of woman who takes the conscious and often difficult steps to ensure that her baby is born at home, who is prepared to take responsibility for her life and for that of her baby, is likely to be the sort of person able to confront the possibility of such a thing occurring.

The following two accounts are from women who did just that. Their stories tell very movingly how they managed when it happened to them, and answer some of the questions raised far more eloquently than I can. Hazel's conveys a very clear impression that Jamie had the best possible start and end to a life that was destined to be very short. It is difficult to believe that hospital care could have been anywhere near so good. It is interesting, but not surprising, that their experiences confirmed Mary and Hazel's belief in home birth.

"I was very happy to find myself pregnant, but it was a strange feeling to find that happiness eroding over the following nine months. Those months leading to the stillbirth of our son Jonathan were very sad. My sense of self slipped away in the face of opposition to my decision to have a home birth, and what gradually seemed like the whole world telling me to do this or that, and that I should feel this way or that way. Having decided on a home birth it was pointed out to me that I was silly, stubborn and thinking only of myself and of course that I was almost encouraging the worst thing of all to happen, the death or stillbirth of our child. Of course nobody really thought that it would happen, save myself, for I often felt that something was wrong and certainly began to feel worthless and useless in the most important role I had ever undertaken. I felt more and more in an unhappy, desperate state of resenting the pregnancy. It seemed a pregnancy for others to deal with, that others wanted and assumed responsibility for, although no one else could assume the emotional responsibility. But sadly I never felt able to reveal to my unborn child the real intimate respect for his unique life that I wanted to; that is, not until he was stillborn.

"Jonathan's stillbirth was a real event, the first family event for my husband and me, although an event full of grief. Our real and only child had died just before being born in our family home. It is sad indeed that in comparing our feelings during the pregnancy with those of Jonathan's stillbirth, the latter felt the more positive experience, one of which my husband and I have deep and even fond memories.

"Our baby remained with us for about an hour and we are glad to have the memory of his presence for that short time in our home. We felt uninhibited in our reactions to the stillbirth, we were not in a strange place with strange people, we were in a place intimate to us and in each other's company – free to hold the baby, look at him, cry, talk and comfort each other. During that short hour the doctor baptised him and we photographed him. I feel that his spiritual presence was recognised in baptism to be destined for God's world, not ours, and that photographing him would give us a memento of his physical presence having touched our world for a while. It is lovely to have his photograph as such an accurate reminder of his face, for without it I would grieve as time dulled my memory. Wrapped in the quilt that I had made for him, he was taken to the pathologist for a post-mortem examination, something I still find hard to think of. It is hard not to think of such a thing as being a mutilation of my baby that looked so perfect and innocent, though still. We chose not to look at him again before his burial.

"During the days that followed I was not confined to bed, and thus I was able to share with my husband the making of the arrangements for a simple funeral service and burial. These arrangements were made with our local priest and the local funeral director. We were sad to hear from the undertaker that few people made the arrangements that we were making. He told us that stillborn babies, if not cremated, were usually buried in the coffin of any adult who had died around that time; sadly, they do not even have the dignity of their own grave to mark their short life. We purchased a child's grave for Jonathan in the Catholic plot of a very attractive local cemetery. In fact we spent many hours looking at cemeteries, for we wanted him to be buried in what we felt a nice place, but settled on a more local cemetery in the end as we also felt it important to be able to visit the grave whenever we wanted to. Purchasing a grave outside one's local district is also much more expensive and complicated to arrange. Jonathan was buried in the purple nightgown which I had made for him before he was born and around his neck hung the cross I had worn during the pregnancy, and a tiny silver ring with his initials inscribed on it. The ring was one of a set of three, the other two being for my husband and myself. We did not want the funeral to be a sombre or formal occasion, preferring a more simple and intimate service for the burial of such an innocent child. We brought flowers from our garden and from friends to lay on the small white coffin. There were only a good friend, the two midwives and ourselves present at the service and graveside, and of course the priest.

"The stillbirth had to be registered and, more so than his funeral, registering his death with my signature had a terrible note of finality. The words on the certificate of stillbirth which I was given by the doctor to present to the registrar are grim words for any mother to read. They are as follows: *'To be given only in respect of a child which has issued forth from its mother after the 28th week of pregnancy and which did not at any time after being completely expelled from its mother, breathe or show any other signs of life.'*

"I remember a feeling of intense anger on first reading these words just after Jonathan was born, anger at such a harsh description of what had just happened. They seemed vulgar words to describe the event of our innocent child passing through our lives. These words also emphasised for us the all too easy feeling to develop, that the rest of the world did not think of Jonathan as having been a human being as unique as you or me. There is no place for his name on the certificate of stillbirth and the chosen name for a stillborn child is only put on the register of birth and deaths if you request it to be there.

I feel sure that because I was able to experience Jonathan's birth in the way that I did, seeing him and holding him and arranging for his burial myself, I never faced the problems that some women have after a stillbirth of never being able to look after other babies. I knew how unique Jonathan was; there would never be a need to compare.

"Our experience, though sad, was rewarding in our lives. Just as many feel rewarded with a healthy baby, so we had the opportunity and fortune to feel rewarded in many different ways by Jonathan.

"I became pregnant again six months after Jonathan was born and had a marvellous pregnancy, in as much isolation from the world and doctors as I could achieve. I was determined simply to enjoy the pregnancy, for I knew this would help my conviction that it would be a healthy pregnancy and all would be well at the birth. I arranged another home birth, but virtually never felt daunted by the thoughts of labour and the possible outcome. We had experienced one of the worst things that can happen at childbirth in any place of birth, but felt sure that if our second child were to be stillborn, home is where we wanted to be. David was born a very healthy child, at home."

Mary Cooper

"When I first visited my GP I hadn't made up my mind whether to have my baby in hospital or at home. My GP wasn't keen on my having a home birth, but he didn't say anything that convinced me that hospital was safer for the baby. I read as much as I could find on the subject and decided that if my pregnancy was straightforward then I'd have my baby at home. I am the type of person who can bear pain better than embarrassment and I warmed to the idea of giving birth in my own surroundings, in privacy, with just help from my husband and one or two midwives.

"My antenatal care was shared between my GP and the large local hospital. I dreaded the hospital visits, and if I'd had any doubts about having my baby at home those visits certainly dispelled them. The first visit was the worst. The main disagreement we had with the obstetrician was that he wanted me to have a routine scan and I didn't want one. Paul and I had already talked about what I'd do if there was something wrong with the baby and decided it was better if I didn't have a scan, partly because I'm not 100 per cent sure that they're safe and partly because I didn't want to be faced with the decision of whether to have a disabled child aborted or not. The obstetrician just couldn't accept our views and in the end we left. I was shaken and close to tears and only trudged back to the hospital because I thought it was best for the baby.

"My GP arranged for me to have a different consultant, and he was certainly more pleasant. There was one occasion, though, when he said to us 'You feel now that you'd like a home birth, but how will you feel if the baby dies?' Paul answered him firmly, and after that the obstetrician didn't refer to me having a home birth again. As a compromise I agreed to have a scan near the end of my pregnancy. The baby seemed fine with the head well engaged.

"Eventually, a week overdue, I went into labour. What I'd thought were wind pains gradually became a steady mild pain. I had a show, but didn't call the midwives until the next day when the pain increased a little and I could feel my muscles tightening and contracting.

"The midwives came and sorted out the room our baby was to be born in. They brought in an amazing amount of equipment and as they arranged the room, there was an air of excitement about the house. We lived with my mother and this was to be her first grandchild. After the death of my father she had been pretty depressed, but as my pregnancy continued she'd become much happier, going to the hairdressers and buying the occasional new outfit, etc. As the pain was so mild the midwives went away, saying that they'd be back about 11 pm as it didn't look as if anything was going to happen for a while.

"My mother's house backs on to the River Ness and in the middle of the river are two islands accessible by bridges. Paul and I spent that beautiful summer's evening walking the dogs through the islands, imagining that the next time we walked there we would have with us a baby son or daughter.

"By the time we got home the pain was extremely bad and Paul phoned the midwives straight away. They arrived in next to no time and found I was already 8 cm dilated. Eventually one of the midwives ruptured the membranes because I'd been fully dilated for quite some time and in a lot of pain, but had no feeling of wanting to push. There seemed to be pints of amniotic fluid and then nothing. No pain, no contractions and still no urge to push. I stayed like that for about an hour, then one of the midwives said that I should really start to push because I couldn't stay like that indefinitely. This I did. I found that when I squatted and pushed the compulsion to carry on pushing was very strong and I could feel the baby moving. Yet whenever I rested, the desire to push vanished completely. On examining me the midwife realised that the baby's face was coming first instead of the head, and so, just before the birth, she gave me an episiotomy, thinking, understandably, that the head would make a difficult delivery. I remember the episiotomy was excruciatingly painful, then my baby being born and hearing the midwife say, 'I'm sorry, but your baby's not going to live.'

"I could feel the atmosphere, that something was terribly wrong, and then as I went to look, Paul was crying, covering my eyes and holding me. I had to push him away. I wanted to see my baby. I was very confused. Surely if the baby was alive something could be done to help prevent it from dying? Then I looked at him and knew that what the midwife had said was true. He wasn't going to live. He was large, he was very strong, a good colour, but most of his head was missing. It broke my heart to know that it was better that he should die. I said 'He's a boy' and started to cry. Paul and I were hugging each other for comfort. The midwives wrapped Jamie up warmly and I held him. Paul asked how long he was likely to live and I felt shocked when the midwives said just an hour or two. I somehow had thought he would live for a few weeks or months. I felt panic rising in me. He was going to die before we'd even got a chance to know each other. The overriding feeling I had was that he must be cuddled and loved whilst he lived. I wanted him to know that just because he wasn't perfect that didn't alter the fact that we loved him. I didn't want him to be on his own, and I was particularly worried when the doctor came to stitch me that he might die on his own in the cot. I felt very relieved when I saw one of the midwives pick him up and walk up and down with him. From then on, someone always held him.

"Paul had the sad job of going downstairs and breaking the news to my mother. She then came up to meet Jamie. Paul also phoned his father who was also eagerly awaiting the birth of his first grandchild. I felt guilty that I'd let so many people down – Paul, my mother, my brother, my father-in-law, the midwives, and most of all Jamie himself.

"Our GP spoke to us for a while, basically saying what many people were to say to us later; that we could have more babies, etc. I felt like screaming 'I don't want more babies, I want this one!' But we were very polite and thanked him. The poor man didn't mean to be unkind, he was upset and didn't really know what to say. He told my mother that he hadn't wanted me to have a home birth, but under the circumstances it was better that Jamie was born at home, because in hospital he would have been taken away and put in an incubator and I probably wouldn't have seen him.

"Jamie, instead of just living an hour or two, lived for almost three days. All the time we held him, spoke to him and gently stroked his cheek. After our initial shock, when we could only see what was wrong with him, we began to see everything that was perfect about him. He had such a lovely face. He looked very like Paul. His body was so strong and what a grip his fingers had! Friends called to see him. Although we are not churchgoers, the minister who had married us came to see us, and spoke a great deal of sense, advising us not to rush into another pregnancy in the hope of replacing Jamie, but to take time to grieve for Jamie after he had died. He also said what I believe to be true; that it was love that was keeping Jamie alive. My brother and Paul's father drove up from London together in time to spend a few hours with Jamie and I know that meeting him meant a great deal to both of them. The obstetrician also called at the house. I think he must have felt a little guilty because he stressed that Jamie's condition had nothing to do with the fact that he was born at home. He also explained that the scan hadn't shown Jamie's condition up because it just appeared as if his head had been well engaged. A scan earlier in my pregnancy would most probably have shown Jamie's condition.

"Our doctor (and later on all the medical textbooks I could find) say that anencephalic babies can't feel anything because their brain hasn't formed. But we began to realise that Jamie could feel. His responses weren't just reflexes, he responded to us. For instance he started to whimper when we put him down on a towel to change his nappy; then, when he felt the warm water he quietened, smiling and calm. One night when both my mother and Paul were asleep, I lay down with Jamie lying in the crook of my arm, and with my other hand stroked his cheek. I was so tired that I kept falling asleep, but each time I drifted off, Jamie woke me by fidgeting and shuffling, making little noises, until I started to stroke his cheek again, whereupon he immediately relaxed again.

"On Saturday at 8.30 pm Jamie started having convulsions and finally died at 11.25 pm. He was very distressed during these convulsions and all we could do was hold him, tell him we loved him, but he must give in and die now. It was such a relief when the convulsions stopped and he died. He was at peace. Very quietly and methodically we bathed him and dried him. We looked through all the clothes we'd bought for him and chose a pretty white flannelette nightdress to dress him in. This was the first and only time we dressed him. We wrapped him in a lace shawl so that his head was covered but his beautiful face showed. We put clean sheets on his cot and laid him down on it. Then as a final touch we laid a pink carnation beside him. Perhaps to an outsider this sounds morbid, but we felt pleased to be able to do one more thing for him. When we'd finished we went downstairs to tell the others that he was dead and they each went up to say goodbye to him on their own.

"All the doctors in the practice knew that Jamie's death was imminent but when Paul phoned, the doctor who took the call asked the time of death and then snapped angrily that it was now 1.00 am and what had taken us so long to phone? Paul told him not to bother coming round and we would see our own GP the next day.

"We kept Jamie's body in our room until he was buried the following Tuesday. The funeral director put him into a small white coffin, but didn't alter the way we'd dressed and arranged him. I liked having him there for those few extra days, just being able to look at him. It made his going just a little more gradual and gave us a little longer to say goodbye. After his funeral the room seemed so empty and that really was the hard part to come to terms with. At least we had our memories of him and some treasured photographs, and of course each other.

"Looking back, four and a half years later, I'm so pleased I had Jamie at home. Not just for myself, but I think for everyone, including Jamie; the home environment was best for us. My one regret is that I didn't breastfeed him. I knew he wanted to feed and on the third day I gave him a bottle with water to drink. I think to start with I didn't feed him because I was expecting him to die at any moment; then when I did begin to think of feeding him no one suggested I should and I thought perhaps there was something 'improper' about me wanting to feed a baby who was going to die. Also I was very clumsy and inexperienced with him. I'd never even held a baby before, but I regret not following my instincts.

"On a happier note we now have two healthy boys, Ruairi who is two and a half and Thomas who is nine months old. Both were born at home, and what happy occasions their births were. After my experiences at the hospital I had all my antenatal care with my GP or the community midwives. Because there is a 1 in 20 chance of my having another baby with a neural tube defect I knew the hospital would be very keen on my having various tests, and I just didn't want any more arguments. I had to find another GP because the one I had decided to strike me off his list for wanting another home birth. He felt women should be able to have home births, but he didn't want to be involved. One of my midwives helped me to find a doctor who was willing to take me (and the rest of my family) on. It is extremely difficult to have a home birth in this part of the country, but unless there is a particular reason for having to go into hospital, I would prefer to have my babies at home."

Hazel Johnston

14 rest after the birth

There is a disadvantage to having a baby at home – namely the expectation that, because you have not been in hospital, you are able to continue an active life without a rest. If you are at home you are available to solve any housekeeping or childcare problem. You are also available to visitors, who are unrestricted by visiting hours.

You may feel wonderfully fit after having a baby at home. You are less likely to have had drugs or an episiotomy, or for your labour to have been induced or accelerated. You may not have had syntometrine and your labour may have been shorter than if it had been in hospital. All these things can contribute to your feeling as if you can carry on just where you left off. However this does not mean that you should. Your body has undergone huge physiological changes, and you need time and space to establish feeding, to get to know your new baby as an individual and to rest and recover. After an initial period of sleepiness, the baby is likely to want frequent feeding, both day and night. This lasts at least for several weeks, if not months, and you will feel better if you get a chance to rest in the earliest days.

There is currently no great respect in our society for the postnatal period. In other cultures it is seen as a special time, when a mother should be freed from the obligations of work and domestic routine in order to recover quietly and learn to love and look after her new baby. This period varies from three or four days to 90, with nine or ten apparently being common. It used to be common practice in this country for a woman to 'lie in' (in bed) for a month following her confinement (this was so well-recognised that in the seventeenth century parishes paid for unmarried mothers to lie in, even though they were very reluctant to accept the collective responsibility for the care of fatherless children). Nowadays the length of stay in hospital, even following Caesarean section, which is a major operation, may only be three days. The consequence of financial cuts in the National Health Service can mean a maximum hospital stay of one or two days, even with a first baby. This leads women to feel that it is expected of them that they are up and active soon after the birth, regardless of the fact that the baby now has to be fed externally rather than internally and that the amount of milk you can offer a baby depends on your having enough energy to produce it.

There is a Chinese medical belief that a woman should spend ten days in bed following the birth of her child. This means that the risk of her getting postnatal depression is greatly reduced.[42] This distressing illness is in any case less common in women having their babies at home, but it does seem to make sense to stay in bed for that period of time and have things done for you. For many women it is the only time that they do get a break from domestic routine. If you have only recently given up work it may be even more important to take time over the transition to motherhood. There is also evidence to suggest that failure to rest while your uterus returns to its pre-pregnancy size and shape will predispose you to uterine prolapse in later life. This may seem too remote to worry about, but is something you will certainly regret if it does occur. You really don't get any marks for going running the day that your baby is born.

How you can help yourself

It is vital that you have someone with you in your home to prepare meals, do the washing, answer the door and phone, take the children to school or entertain them while you are asleep, and take the baby off your hands while you rest. This might be your partner, mother or mother-in-law, sister or friend, but it is important that they are prepared to do the job and will not be combining it with work, or only popping in occasionally.

- Have as many prepared meals in the freezer as possible, for the days following the postnatal period.
- Make sure that you eat and drink well.
- Make sure that you have the midwives' number in case you or the baby need help. They are on call 24 hours a day if you need them.

- The midwife will bath your baby initially if you choose. If you have not done it before, wait until you feel strong before starting. Babies don't need bathing every day.
- Enjoy the postpartum period and try and relax and rest – ideally with you both in bed – the baby just in a nappy and you just in pants and pad. It really is a very short time and there will be plenty of time for everything else later.

Visitors may be welcome, provided you see them while you are in bed and they or your helper make the tea. If they are staying too long, or expect you to look after them, you will have to insist on restricted visiting hours. The following account, by a first-time mother of a baby born at home, shows why.

"Another time, and given a bit more lead-in time [she changed her booking 12 days before she was due], I would have built in more support for ourselves after the birth. It resulted in Dave doing what the hospital staff do so well – taking care of all the practical needs of mother and baby, feeding, washing, shopping, cooking, etc. which is a great demand on top of being a new parent.

"Also, the regulated visiting hours at hospital are, on reflection, a boon; adjusting and coping with the enormity of a new baby is tiring to say the least. It is much more challenging to structure 'visiting hours' when you have a home birth, and delighted friends want to call by at odd hours to share in the celebration. After a week of what seemed like non-stop visits, Dave and I finally put the shutters up to all visitors for a couple of weeks, to give ourselves a chance. It was hard to do, but essential."

Vanessa Helps

She echoes my sentiments when she concludes:

"What I have discovered is that if you really want a home birth, you can get it. Expect and welcome the upheaval it will cause. There will be many people who will be right behind what you are aiming for, including medical staff and midwives and particularly me!"

references

1. *Where can I have my baby?* www.nhsdirect.nhs.uk
2. NICE (National Institute for Health and Clinical Excellence) draft guidelines, June 2006.
3. Patricia Hewitt, Department of Health, May 15 2006 'wants to end the assumption that hospital is always the best place to have a baby', www.bbc.co.uk.
4. Campbell, R. and A. Macfarlane, *Where To Be Born?*, National Perinatal Epidemiology Unit, 1995.
5. *Midwives Chronicle*, July 1992, 167-74.
6. *Health Committee Maternity Services Report*, HMSO, 1992.
7. Changing Childbirth Part I. Report of the Expert Maternity Group. Part II Survey of Good Communication in Practice, HMSO, 1993.
8. Department of Health. National Service Framework for Children, Young People and Maternity Services – Maternity. 2004. London, Department of Health.
9. Lederman, R.P., E. Lederman, B.A. Work and D.S. McCann, 'The relationship of maternal anxiety plasma catechelomine in plasma cortisol to progress in labour', *Am. J. Obstet. Gynec.* 132 (1978): 495-500; E. Lederman, R.P. Lederman, B.A. Work and D.S. McCann, 'Maternal, psychological and physiological correlates of fetal newborn health status', *Am. J. Obstet. Gynec.* 139 (1981): 956-8; Burns, J.K., 'Relationship between blood levels of cortisol and duration of human labour', *J. Physiol.* 254 (1976): 12.
10. Morse, J.M. and C. Park, 'Homebirth and hospital deliveries: a comparison of the perceived painfulness of parturition', *Nursing and Health* (Edmonton, Alberta) 11, no. 3 (1988): 175-81.
11. Stillwell, J.A., 'Relative costs of home and hospital confinement', *B.M.J.*, 1979: 257-9.
12. Postnatal infection survey, National Childbirth Trust, 1987.
13. Damastra-Wijmenja, S.M.I., 'Home confinement: the positive results in Holland', *Journ. Royal Coll. Gen. Pract.* 34 (1984): 425-30; Treffers, P.E., and R. Laan, 'Regional perinatal mortality and regional hospitalisation at delivery in the Netherlands', *British Journal of Obstetrics and*

Gynaecology. (July 1986): 690-3.
14. *Midwifery Today*, www.midwiferytoday.com/enews, January 18, 2006, Vol 8, Issue 2.
15. Chiswick, M., 'Intrauterine growth retardation', *B.M.J.* 291, 1985, 845-8; Hall, M.H., P.K. Chung and I. Macgillivray, 'Is routine antenatal care worthwhile?', *Lancet* 1980: 78-80.
16. Augensen, Kare, Per Bergsjo, Torunn Eikeland, Kjell Ashvik and Johannes Carlsen, 'Randomised comparison of early versus late induction of labour in postterm pregnancy', *B.M.J.* 294, 9 May 1987: 1192-5; Gibbs, D,M.F., L.D. Cardozo, J.W.W. Studd and D.J. Cooper, 'Prolonged pregnancy; is induction of labour indicated?', *Br. Journ. Obs. and Gynaec.*, 1982: 292-5.
17. Shearer, J.M.L., 'Five year prospective study of risk of booking for a home birth', *B.M.J.* 291, 1985: 1478-80. A comparison of 202 home births compared with 185 births in a consultant unit found double the induction rate, a higher rate of episiotomies, second degree tears and more babies with low Apgar scores in the hospital group.
18. Prentice, A., and T. Lind, 'Continuous fetal heart rate monitoring', *Lancet*, 12 December 1987: 1375-7.
19. Caldeyro-Barcia, R., 'Possible iatrogenic effects of rupture of the membrane during fetal monitoring'. In *Perinatale Medizin*, edited by J.W. Dudenhausen and E. Sating, Stuttgart, Georg Thieme Verlag, 1975.
20. Hannah M.E., W.J. Hannah, S.A. Hewson, F.D. Hodnett, S. Saigal, and A.R. Willan, 'Planned caesarean section versus planned vaginal birth for breech presentation at term: a randomised multicentre trial'. Term Breech Collaborative Group. *Lancet* 2000 Oct 21; 356(9239): 1375-83. See also Royal College of Midwives critique at www.rcmnormal-birth.org.uk.
21. Allison, Julia, 'Midwives step out of the shadows', *Midwives Chronicle* (July 1992): 167-79.
22. Myers, Stephen, A., and Norbert Gleichen, 'Breech delivery: why the dilemma?', *Am. J. Obstet. and Gynec.* 156 (January 1987): 6-10.
23. Nwosu, E.C., S. Walkinshaw, P. Chia, and others, *British Journal of Obstetrics and Gynaecology*, vol 100, no 6, June 1993: 531-5.
24. Skibsted, L. and A. P. Lange, 'The need for pain relief in uncomplicated deliveries in an alternative birth centre compared to an obstetric delivery ward', *Pain*, vol 48, no 2, February 1992: 183-6.
25. Paper presented at the International Confederation of Midwives, 21st Congress, The Hague, August 1988; Leslie Ludka, Midwives Information and Resource Service pack, April 1988.
26. Shuman, A.N., and T.M. Marteau, 'Obstetricians' and midwives' contrasting perceptions of pregnancy', *Journal of Reproductive and Infant Psychology*, vol 11, no 2, April 1993: 115-18.
27. NHS Direct.

28. Nursing and Midwifery Council circular, 2006-8. The circular runs to four pages and can be seen at www.nmc-uk.org.
29. Gastaldo, T.D. (correspondence), *Birth*, vol 19, no 4, December 1992: 230.
30. Junor, V. and M. Monaco, *The Home Birth Handbook*, Souvenir Press, 1984.
31. Garrey, Matthew, A.D.T. Govan, Colin Hodge and R. Callander, *Obstetrics Illustrated*, Churchill Livingstone, 1980.
32. Cardozo, L., 'Is routine induction of labour at term ever justified?' *British Medical Journal*, vol 306, no 6881, 27 March 1993: 840-1.
33. NICE (National Institute for Health and Clinical Excellence) draft guidelines, June 2006.
34. Allot, H.A., and C.R. Palmer, 'Sweeping the membranes: a valid procedure in stimulating the onset of labour?' *British Journal of Obstetrics and Gynaecology*, vol 100, no 10, Oct 1993: 898-903; Grant, J.M, 'Sweeping the membranes in prolonged pregnancy', *British Journal of Obstetrics and Gynaecology*, vol 100, no 10, Oct 1993: 889-90.
35. Beckwith, J. and M. Read, *British Journal of Midwifery*, Feb 1996, vol 4, no 2.
36. Duncan, S. and S. Beckley, 'The evidence from an obstetric point of view is summarised in prelabour rupture of the membranes – why hurry?' *British Journal of Obstetrics and Gynaecology*, vol 99, no 7, July 1992: 543-5.
37. Brown, Lyn. 'The tide has turned: Audit of water birth', *British Journal of Midwifery*, April 1998, Vol 6, No 4, pp 236-243.
38. NICE (National Institute for Health and Clinical Excellence) draft guidelines, June 2006, 1.6.7.
39. Katz, V.L. and W.A. Bowes, 'Meconium aspiration syndrome: reflections on a murky subject', *American Journal of Obstetrics and Gynaecology*, vol 166, no 1, January 1992: 171-83.
40. Johnson K.C. and B.A. Daviss 'Outcomes of planned home births with certified professional midwives: large prospective study in North America'. *BMJ* 2005; 330 (7505): 141 ; Woodcock H.C., A.W. Read, C. Bower, F.J. Stanley and D.J Moore, 'A matched cohort study of planned home and hospital births in Western Australia 1981-1987', *Midwifery* 1994; 10(3): 125-135.; Woodcock H.C., A.W. Read, D.J. Moore, F.J Stanley and C. Bower, 'Planned home births in Western Australia 1981-1987: a descriptive study', *Med J Aust* 1990; 153 (11-12): 672-8.
41. Gaskin, Ina May, 'Shoulder dystocia: controversies in management', *The Birth Gazette* 5 (Fall 1988): 14-17.
42. The Association for Post-natal Illness, www.apni.org.

All the references used by NICE in drafting the guidelines for intrapartum care (June 2006) are available in the report. A selection of the research particularly relating to home birth includes:

Ackermann-Liebrich U, Voegeli T, Gunter-Witt K, Kunz I, Zullig M, Schindler C et al. 'Home versus hospital deliveries: Follow up study of matched pairs for procedures and outcome', *BMJ* 1996.

Bastian H, Keirse MJ, Lancaster PA. 'Perinatal death associated with planned home birth in Australia: population based study', *BMJ* 1998.

Davies J, Hey E, Reid W, Young G. 'Prospective regional study of planned home births', *BMJ* 1996.

Caplan M, Madeley RJ. 'Home deliveries in Nottingham 1980-81', Public Health 1985.

Chamberlain G, Wraight A, Crowley P. 'Home births – The report of the 1994 Confidential Enquiry by the National Birthday Trust Fund', Parthenon; 1997.

Collaborative survey of perinatal loss in planned and unplanned home births. Northern Region Perinatal Mortality Survey Coordinating Group. *BMJ* 1996.

Duran AM. 'The safety of home birth: the farm study', *Am J Public Health* 1992.

Ford C, Iliffe S, Franklin O. 'Outcome of planned home births in an inner city practice', *BMJ* 1991.

Janssen PA, Lee SK, Ryan EM, Etches DJ, Farquharson DF, Peacock D et al. 'Outcomes of planned home births versus planned hospital births after regulation of midwifery in British Columbia', *Can Med Assoc J* 2002.

Johnson KC, Daviss BA. 'Outcomes of planned home births with certified professional midwives: large prospective study in North America', *BMJ* 2005.

Macfarlane A, Mugford M. 'Birth Counts: Statistics of pregnancy & childbirth', Volume 1. 2 ed. London: The Stationary Office; 2000.

Mehl LE. 'Research on alternatives in childbirth: what can it tell us about hospital practice?' In: Stewart L, Stewart D, editors. 21st century obstetrics now. Marble Hill, MO: NAPSAC; 1977.

Olsen O, Jewell MD. Home versus hospital birth. Cochrane Database of Systematic Reviews [1]. 2005.

Olsen O. Meta-analysis of the Safety of Home Birth. *Birth* 1997

Standing Maternity and Midwifery Advisory Committee. Domiciliary midwifery and maternity beds needed. 1970. London, HMSO.

Tew M. 'Safer childbirth: a critical history of maternity care', 3rd edition ed. London: Free Association Books Ltd; 1998.

Welsh Assembly Government. National Service Framework for Children, Young People and Maternity Services in Wales. 2005.

Wiegers TA, Keirse MJ, van der ZJ, Berghs GA. 'Outcome of planned home and planned hospital births in low risk pregnancies: prospective study in midwifery practices in The Netherlands', *BMJ* 1996.

further reading

Janet Balaskas, *New Active Birth*, Collins, 1990
Beverley Lawrence Beech, *Choosing a Home Birth*, AIMS
Abigail Cairns, *Home Births: Stories to Inspire and Inform*, Lonely Scribe, 2006
Rona Campbell and **Alison Macfarlane**, *Where to be Born?*, National Perinatal Epidemiology Unit, 1995
Jean Donnison, *Midwives and Medical Men*, Historical Publications, 1988
Nadine Pilley Edwards, *Birthing Autonomy: Women's Experiences of Planning Home Births*, Routledge, 2005
Nadine Pilley Edwards and **Beverly Lawrence Beech**, *Birthing Your Baby: The Second Stage*, AIMS 2001
Ina May Gaskin, *Ina May's Guide to Childbirth*, Bantam 2003
Henci Goer, *The Thinking Woman's Guide to a Better Birth*, Perigee Books, 1999
Sally Inch, *Birthrights: Parents' Guide to Modern Childbirth*, Green Print, 1989
Margaret Jowitt, *Childbirth Unmasked*, Peter Wooller, 1993
Viki Junor and **Marianne Monaco**, *The Home Birth Handbook*, Souvenir Press, 1984
Sheila Kitzinger, *The Politics of Birth*, Books for Midwives, 2005
Nicky Leap and **Billie Hunter**, *The Midwife's Tale: An Oral History from Handywoman to Professional Midwife*, Scarlet Press, 1993
Anna McGrail and **Daphne Metland**, *Expecting: Everything you need to know about pregnancy, labour and birth*, Virago Press, 2004
Ann Oakley, **Ann McPherson** and **Helen Roberts**, *Miscarriage*, Penguin, 1990
Camilla Palmer, *Maternity and Parental Rights: A Parent's Guide to Rights at Work*, Legal Action Group, 2006

Angela Phillips, **Barbara Jacobs** and **Nicky Lean**, *Your Body, Your Baby, Your Life: Guide to Pregnancy and Childbirth*, Pandora Press, 1983

Andrea Robertson, *Empowering Women*, Birth International, 1999

Marjorie Tew, *Safer Childbirth? A Critical History of Maternity Care*, Free Association Books, 1998

Nancy Warner Cohen and **Lois J. Esther**, *Silent Knife: Cesarean Prevention and Vaginal Birth After Cesarean*, Greenwood, 1983

Nicky Wesson, *Alternative Maternity*, Vermilion, 1996

Nicky Wesson, *Labour Pain*, Healing Arts Press, 2000

Sarah Wickham, *Induction – Do I Really Need It?*, AIMS, 2004

Sarah Wickham, *What's Right For Me? Making Decisions in Pregnancy and Birth*, AIMS, 2002

Kim Wildner, *Mother's Intention: How Belief Shapes Birth*, Harbor & Hill, 2003

for children

Jenni Overend and **Julie Vivas**, *Hello Baby*, Francis Lincoln, 2004

Uwe Spillman, *Runa's Birth: The Day My Sister Was Born*, Made in Water, 2006

useful addresses*

Acupuncture

The British Acupuncture Council
63 Jeddo Road, London W12 9HQ, Tel 020 8735 0400
info@acupuncture.org.uk, **www.acupuncture.org.uk**
Register of acupuncturists.

AcuMedic
101-105 Camden High Street, London NW1 7JN, Tel 020 7388 5783
info@acumedic.com, **www.acumedic.com**
Shop selling books about acupuncture, moxa, needles, etc.
Clinic 7 days a week, by appointment only.

Bach flower remedies

The Dr Edward Bach Centre
Mount Vernon, Bakers Lane, Brightwell-cum-Sotwell, Oxon OX10 0PZ, UK
Tel 01491 834678
www.bachcentre.com

Chiropractic

British Chiropractic Association
59 Castle Street, Reading, Berkshire RG1 7SN, Tel 0118 950 5950
Provides list of qualified chiropractors.
enquiries@chiropractic-uk.co.uk, **www.chiropractic-uk.co.uk**

Complementary medicine

Foundation for Integrated Health
33-41 Dallington Street, London EC1V 0BB, Tel 020 3119 3100
info@fih.org.uk, **www.fih.org.uk**

* for regularly updated useful addresses and links see the publisher's
website at **www.pinterandmartin.com**

The Research Council for Complementary and Alternative Medicine
www.rccm.org.uk

Institute of Complementary Medicine
ICM PO Box 194, London SE16 7QZ, Tel 020 7237 5165
info@i-c-m.org.uk, **www.i-c-m.org.uk**
Provides a list of practitioners.

Homeopathy

British Homeopathy Association
Hahnemann House, 29 Park Street West, Luton LU1 3BE, Tel 0870 444 3950
www.trusthomeopathy.org
Will supply a list of medically qualified doctors who are also qualified in
homeopathy and pharmacists stocking homeopathic medicines.

The Society of Homeopaths
11 Brookfield, Duncan Close, Moulton Park, Northampton NN3 6WL,
Tel 0845 450 6611
info@homeopathy-soh.org, **www.homeopathy-soh.org**
Will supply a list of registered homeopaths.

Hypnotherapy

British Hypnotherapy Association
67 Upper Berkeley Street, London W1H 7QX, Tel 020 7723 4443
www.hypnotherapy-association.org

British Society of Medical and Dental Hypnosis
28 Dale Park Gardens, Cookridge, Leeds LS16 7PT, Tel 07000 560309
www.bsmdh.org

Reflexology

The Association of Reflexologists
5 Fore Street, Taunton, Somerset, TA1 1HX, Tel 0870 5673320
www.aor.org.uk
Search for practitioners.

Medical herbalism

National Institute of Medical Herbalists
Elm House, 54 Mary Arches Street, Exeter EX4 3BA, Tel 01392 426022
nimh@ukexeter.freeserve.co.uk, **www.nimh.org.uk**
For a list of practitioners.

The College of Practitioners of Phytotherapy
Oak Glade, 9 Hythe Close, Polegate, BN26 6LQ, Tel 01323 484353
pamela.bull@btopenworld.com, **www.phytotherapists.org**

Osteopathy

General Osteopathic Council
176 Tower Bridge Road, London, SE1 3LU, Tel 020 7357 6655
info@osteopathy.org.uk, **www.osteopathy.org.uk**
List of registered osteopaths.

Cranial therapy

Craniosacral Therapy Association
Monomark House, 27 Old Gloucester Street, London WC1N 3XX
Tel 07000 784 735
office@craniosacral.co.uk, **www.craniosacral.co.uk**

General health

Action on Pre-Eclampsia (APEC)
84-88 Pinner Road, Harrow HA1 4HZ, Tel 020 8863 3271
info@apec.org.uk, **www.apec.org.uk**

Action for Sick Children
36 Jacksons Edge Road, Disley, Stockport, SK12 2JL, Tel 0800 0744519
www.actionforsickchildren.org

Active Birth Centre
25 Bickerton Road London N19 5JT, Tel 020 7281 6760
info@activebirthcentre.com, **www.activebirthcentre.com**

AIMS – Association for Improvements in the Maternity Services
5 Ann's Court, Grove Road, Surbiton KT6 4BE, Tel 0870 765 1433
www.aims.org.uk

Antenatal Results and Choices
73 Charlotte Street, London W1T 4PN, Tel 020 7631 0285
info@arc-uk.org, **www.arc-uk.org**

Association of Breastfeeding Mothers
PO Box 207, Bridgwater, Somerset TA6 7YT, Tel 0870 401 7711
info@abm.me.uk, **www.abm.me.uk**

Association for Postnatal Illness
145 Dawes Road, Fulham, London SW6 7EB, Tel 020 7386 0868
info@apni.org, **www.apni.org**

Association of Radical Midwives
16 Wytham Street, Oxford OX1 4SU, Tel 01865 248159
www.radmid.demon.co.uk

Campaign for Normal Birth
www.rcmnormalbirth.org.uk

Caesarean.org.uk
Caesarean and VBAC information including home birth after Caesarean.
www.caesarean.org.uk

Cry-sis
BM Cry-sis, London WC1N 3XX, 08451 228 669
info@cry-sis.org.uk, www.cry-sis.org.uk
Help with crying babies.

Down's Syndrome Association
Langdon Down Centre, 2a Langdon Park, Teddington TW11 9PS. Tel 0845
230 0372
info@downs-syndrome.org.uk, www.downs-syndrome.org.uk

Doula UK
PO Box 26678, London, N14 4WB, Tel 0871 433 3103
info@doula.org.uk, www.doula.org.uk

Foresight – Association for the Promotion of Preconceptual Care
178 Hawthorn Road, West Bognor PO21 2UY, Tel 01243 868001
www.foresight-preconception.org.uk

The Foundation for the Study of Infant Deaths
Artillery House, 11-19 Artillery Row, London SW1P 1RT
Helpline: 020 7233 2090, General: 020 7222 8001
fsid@sids.org.uk, www.sids.org.uk

Gingerbread – the organisation for lone parent families
307 Borough High Street, London SE1 1JH, Tel 020 7403 9500
advice@gingerbread.org.uk, www.gingerbread.org.uk

Homebirth.org.uk
Homebirth reference site with much information and many links.
www.homebirth.org.uk

Independent Midwives Association
89 Green Lane, Farncombe GU7 3TB, Tel 01483 425833
information@independentmidwives.org.uk, www.independentmid-wives.org.uk

La Leche League (Great Britain)
PO Box 29, West Bridgford, Nottingham, NG2 7NP, Tel 0845 456 1855
admin@laleche.org.uk, **www.laleche.org.uk**
Breastfeeding advice.

London Hazards Centre
Hampstead Town Hall Centre, 213 Haverstock Hill, London NW3 4QP, Tel
020 7794 5999
mail@lhc.org.uk, **www.lhc.org.uk**
Advice on occupational hazards in pregnancy.

MAMA – The Meet-a-mum Association
54 Lillington Road, Radstock BA3 3NR, Tel 0845 120 3746
www.mama.co.uk

MIDIRS – Midwives Information and Resource Service
9 Elmdale Road, Clifton, Bristol BS8 1SL, Tel 0800 581 009
www.midirs.org

The Miscarriage Association
c/o Clayton Hospital, Northgate, Wakefield WF1 3JS, Tel 01924 200799
info@miscarriageassociation.org.uk, **www.miscarriageassociation.org.uk**

NCT (National Childbirth Trust)
Alexandra House, Oldham Terrace, London W3 6NH, Tel 0870 770 3236
enquiries@nct.org.uk, **www.nctpregnancyandbabycare.com**

National Child Minding Association
Royal Court, 81 Tweedy Road, Bromley BR1 1TG, Tel 0845 880 0044
info@ncma.org.uk, **www.ncma.org.uk**

National Council for One Parent Families
255 Kentish Town Road, London NW5 2LX, Tel 020 7428 5400
info@oneparentfamilies.org.uk, **www.oneparentfamilies.org.uk**

National Association for Mental Illness
Tel 0845 7660163
www.mind.org.uk

National Perinatal Epidemiology Unit
University of Oxford, Old Road Campus, Oxford OX3 7LF, Tel 01865
289700
www.npeu.ox.ac.uk

Royal College of Midwives
15 Mansfield Street London W1G 9NH, Tel. 020 7312 3535
info@rcm.org.uk, **www.rcm.org.uk**

Sands - Stillbirth and Neonatal Deaths Society
28 Portland Place, London W1B 1LY, Tel 020 7436 5881
helpline@uk-sands.org, **www.uk-sands.org**

VBAC Information and Support (Vaginal Birth after Caesarean)
c/o Caroline Spear, 50 Whiteways, North Bersted, Bognor Regis, PO22
9AS, Tel 01243 868440

Women's Environmental Network
PO Box 30626 London E1 1TZ, Tel 020 7481 9004
info@wen.org.uk, **www.wen.org.uk**

Working Families
1-3 Berry Street, London EC1V 0AA, Tel 020 7253 7243
office@workingfamilies.org.uk, **www.workingfamilies.org.uk**
work-life balance organisation

Suppliers of herbs and essential oils

G. Baldwin and Co
171/173 Walworth Road, London SE17 1RW, Tel 020 7703 5550
sales@baldwins.co.uk, **www.baldwins.co.uk**

Neal's Yard Remedies
Peacemarsh, Gillingham SP8 4EU, Tel 01747 834 600
mail@nealsyardremedies.com, **www.nealsyardremedies.com**

Homeopathic suppliers

Ainsworths
36 New Cavendish Street, London W1G 8UF, Tel 020 7935 5330
www.ainsworths.com

Galen Homeopathics
Llewell Mill, West Stafford, Dorchester DT2 8AN, Tel 01305 263996

Helios Homoeopathic Pharmacy
89-97 Camden Rd, Tunbridge Wells TN1 2QR, Tel 01892 537254
pharmacy@helios.co.uk, **www.helios.co.uk**

A. Nelson and Co Ltd
Broadheath House, 83 Parkside, Wimbledon, London SW19 5LP, Tel 020 8780 4200
pharmacy@nelsonbach.com, **www.nelsonshomoeopathy.co.uk**

Weleda (UK) Ltd
Heanor Road, Ilkeston DE7 8DR, Tel 0115 944 8200
www.weleda.co.uk

index

also from **Pinter & Martin**

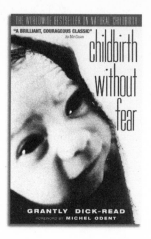

Childbirth without Fear
The Principles and Practice of Natural Childbirth
Grantly Dick-Read
with a foreword by Michel Odent

2004 | paperback | 352 pages | ISBN 978-0-9530964-6-6

In an age where birth has often been overtaken by obstetrics,
Dr Dick-Read's philosophy is still as fresh and relevant as it was
when he originally wrote this book. He unpicks every possible root cause
of western woman's fear and anxiety in pregnancy, childbirth
and breastfeeding and does so with overwhelming heart and empathy.
Essential reading for all parents-to-be, childbirth educators,
midwives and obstetricians!

"When I was heavily pregnant with my first child 25 years ago this
book fell into my hands. That was the start of my belief in natural
childbirth which eventually led to four great births of my own and the
founding of my life's work in the Active Birth Movement.
Grantly Dick-Read's message is inspirational and even more relevant
today than when this book was first published. Every pregnant mother
should read it."

JANET BALASKAS – author of *New Active Birth*

"A brilliant, courageous classic."

INA MAY GASKIN – author of *Ina May's Guide to Childbirth*

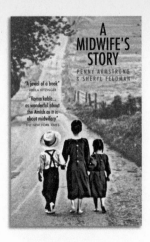

A Midwife's Story
Penny Armstrong & Sheryl Feldman

2006 | paperback | 208 pages | ISBN 978-1-905177-04-2

When hospital-trained midwife Penny Armstrong takes on a job
delivering the babies of the Amish, she encounters a way of life
deeply rooted in the earth. As she renews her respect
for nature she discovers an approach to giving birth
which would change her life for ever.
A gripping first-hand account of Armstrong's journey from student
midwife in Glasgow to running her own practice in rural Pennsylvania,
A Midwife's Story is a life-affirming book that never fails to enlighten, inform
and surprise. Honest and ultimately very moving, it is inspirational reading
not only for midwives and childbirth educators but also for all parents.

"A jewel of a book."
SHEILA KITZINGER

"Remarkable... as wonderful about the Amish as it is about midwifery."
THE NEW YORK TIMES

"Penny Armstrong is a symbol of the revival of midwifery
on the American continent."
MICHEL ODENT – author of Birth Reborn

"Penny Armstrong and Sheryl Feldman have created a loving
and generous book that speaks to many people on many issues:
childbirth, families, the Amish, marriage, deformity, death,
commitment, technology and respect for the land."
ERICA BAUERMEISTER – 500 Great Books by Women

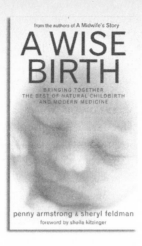

from the authors of A Midwife's Story

A WISE BIRTH

BRINGING TOGETHER
THE BEST OF NATURAL CHILDBIRTH
AND MODERN MEDICINE

penny armstrong & sheryl feldman
foreword by sheila kitzinger

A Wise Birth
Bringing Together the Best of Natural Childbirth and Modern Medicine
Penny Armstrong & Sheryl Feldman
with a foreword by Sheila Kitzinger

2006 | paperback | 240 pages | ISBN 978-1-905177-03-5

What is the best way to give birth to your baby? Is it a hi-tech delivery in a hospital? Or is it more naturally, at home or in a birth centre? Is it possible to combine the best of modern medicine with the non-intervention of natural childbirth?

Penny Armstrong and Sheryl Feldman explore the many issues that influence the way women give birth today: culture and history, technology and psychology. They demonstrate, in a warm and convincing fashion, how to find a setting that will help make your child's birth a healthy and powerful experience.

Informative and provocative, moving and thought-provoking, *A Wise Birth* is based on Penny Armstrong's years of experience as a midwife. It is essential reading for mothers, fathers and childbirth professionals – in fact, anyone interested in the politics of birth.

"Exquisite... *A Wise Birth* speaks eloquently about the uncompromising power of birth."
Mothering

"This thoughtful and well-written book should be read by any and all prospective parents."
Publishers Weekly

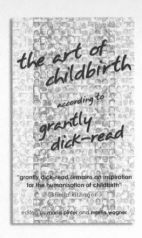

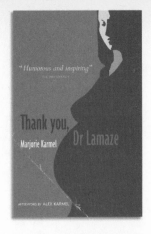

The Art of Childbirth
according to Grantly Dick-Read

ISBN 978-1-905177-01-1

Thank you, Dr Lamaze

ISBN 978-0-9530964-8-0

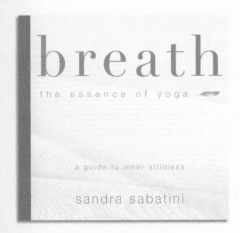

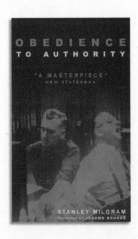

Breath
The Essence of Yoga

ISBN 978-1-905177-09-7

Obedience to Authority

ISBN 978-0-9530964-7-3

visit **www.pinterandmartin.com**
for further information, extracts and special offers